Cooperative Veterinary Care

Cooperative Veterinary Care

Alicea Howell BS, RVT, VTS (Behavior), KPA CTP

Barks and Rec.
Franklin, Indiana, USA

Hillview Veterinary Clinic
Franklin, Indiana, USA

Monique Feyrecilde BA, LVT, VTS (Behavior)

Teaching Animals
Auburn, Washington, USA

Mercer Island Veterinary Clinic
Mercer Island, Washington, USA

WILEY Blackwell

This edition first published 2018
© 2018 John Wiley & Sons, Inc.

The right of Alicea Howell and Monique Feyrecilde to be identified as the authors of this work has been asserted in accordance with law.

Registered Office
John Wiley & Sons, Inc., 111 River Street, Hoboken, NJ 07030, USA

Editorial Office
111 River Street, Hoboken, NJ 07030, USA

For details of our global editorial offices, customer services, and more information about Wiley products visit us at www.wiley.com.

Wiley also publishes its books in a variety of electronic formats and by print-on-demand. Some content that appears in standard print versions of this book may not be available in other formats.

Library of Congress Cataloging-in-Publication Data

Names: Howell, Alicea, 1973– author. | Feyrecilde, Monique, 1977– author.
Title: Cooperative veterinary care / by Alicea Howell, Monique Feyrecilde.
Description: Hoboken, NJ : Wiley, 2018. | Includes bibliographical references and index. |
Identifiers: LCCN 2017040596 (print) | LCCN 2017055417 (ebook) | ISBN 9781119130536 (pdf) |
    ISBN 9781119130543 (epub) | ISBN 9781119130529 (pbk.)
Subjects: LCSH: Veterinary medicine–Practice–Methodology. | MESH: Veterinary Medicine–methods |
    Patient Care–veterinary | Communication | Animal Communication
Classification: LCC SF756.4 (ebook) | LCC SF756.4 .H69 2018 (print) | NLM SF 756.4 |
    DDC 636.089/068–dc23
LC record available at https://lccn.loc.gov/2017040596

Cover Design: Wiley
Cover Image: (Top left and bottom right) Courtesy of Monique Feyrecilde;
(Top right and bottom left) Courtesy of Alicea Howell

Set in 10/12pt Warnock by SPi Global, Pondicherry, India
Printed and bound in Malaysia by Vivar Printing Sdn Bhd

10 9 8 7 6 5 4 3 2 1

Contents

Acknowledgments

Thanks to my husband and true soulmate, Mark, who brings balance and joy to my life.

Thanks to the Doctors, Technicians, and Support Staff, aka "the girls," at Hillview Veterinary Clinic for making this book an everyday reality. You guys are the real deal, and our patients thank you.

Lastly, a special thanks to Dr. Clarke for always giving her technicians space to spread their wings and feel empowered; and to Erin Arvin, aka "Kiki," for your powers of grammar and indexing.

Alicea

I would like to thank my team at Mercer Island Veterinary Clinic for their ongoing support and desire to treat every patient and client with compassion. You feel like family. With your teamwork, my passion became our mission. Every patient, every day benefits from these methods and our desire to treat patients with gentleness and respect. Thank you to Dr. Micah Brodsky for believing in me, for nurturing my ambitions, and for your friendship. Thank you to my wonderful friends for supporting me and this project, and my loyal clients for trusting and allowing me to care for their beloved family members. Thank you, my colleagues and mentors, for elevating the art of veterinary medicine to include the science of learning and behavior.

Most importantly, thank you to my loving and patient husband, Salamandir, without whose support this project would not have been possible. My deepest debt of gratitude is to the animals, who are my most eloquent teachers and among my most treasured companions.

Monique

About the Companion Website

This book is accompanied by a companion website:

www.wiley.com/go/howell/cooperative

There, you will find valuable material designed to enhance your learning, including:

- 108 videos showing procedures described in the book
- All the figures present in the book is available in PowerPoint format for downloading
- Puppy class syllabus
- Puppy Level One homework
- Patient Evaluation and Training Plan Worksheets
- Marketing and Client Education Materials
- Details of Stimulus Control
- Thank-you letters for Alicea Howell and Monique Feyrecilde.

Scan this QR code to visit the companion website.

The videos are clearly signposted throughout the book. Look out for 👁.

1

Introduction to Low-Restraint and No-Restraint Veterinary Care

1.1 First, Do No Harm

Veterinary Technician's Oath
I solemnly dedicate myself to aiding animals and society by providing excellent care and services for animals, **by alleviating animal suffering**, and promoting public health. I accept my obligations to practice my profession conscientiously and with sensitivity, adhering to the profession's Code of Ethics, and furthering my knowledge and competence through a commitment to lifelong learning.

Veterinarian's Oath
I solemnly swear to use my scientific knowledge and skills for the benefit of society through the protection of animal health and **welfare, the prevention and relief of animal suffering**, the conservation of animal resources, the promotion of public health, and the advancement of medical knowledge.

First, do no harm. While these four words do not appear in the oaths, this short sentence certainly describes our mission as health care professionals. Our oath to prevent, relieve, and alleviate animal suffering and the oath's implication of doing no harm apply to both physical and mental or emotional suffering and illnesses of the body. Stress and fear are subjectively harmful and unpleasant on their own, but their physiologic effects of increased heart rate, respiratory rate, blood pressure, temperature, blood glucose levels, cortisol levels, and so many more clearly hold the potential for harm as well.

Recognition and treatment of stress and fear in veterinary patients is not a new concept, but progress is still needed. Dr. Sophia Yin was a pioneer in this field, and her work is still timely and relevant today. She brought the idea of low-stress veterinary care to the mainstream. Dr. Marty Becker has spearheaded the Fear Free[sm] Practice movement in the veterinary profession. We owe thanks to these people and so many more who have come before us, paving the way for this book, which will continue the work of improving veterinary care for patients, clients, and the entire veterinary team. This guide will help the veterinary team take low-stress, compassionate, patient-centered handling to the next level. Mirroring the pediatric model for patient comfort, developing training programs for fearful patients, and embracing the techniques used by progressive zoos and aquariums in their husbandry training programs will all be taught in this guide.

Cooperative Veterinary Care, First Edition. Alicea Howell and Monique Feyrecilde.
© 2018 John Wiley & Sons, Inc. Published 2018 by John Wiley & Sons, Inc.
Companion website: www.wiley.com/go/howell/cooperative

We deserve to take great care of ourselves as well. Veterinary professionals are at high risk for burnout, compassion fatigue, depression, and suicide.[1] Turnover in the veterinary profession is common, with technicians in particular citing burnout. Experiencing stress and potential emotional harm when we are trying to make patients healthy can take a serious toll on veterinary professionals. By using methods that allow patients to relax and cooperate for care, we can make it easier to fulfill our vocation of relieving and preventing animal suffering while keeping our own emotional and mental wellness.

1.2   Stress, Fear, and the Veterinary Clinic

Stress is how the body reacts to a challenge, or stressor. This response is necessary for life. The fear response is a self-protective mechanism that prompts an animal to flee, fight, hide, or react in another helpful way to defend its own safety and well-being. **Fear** and **anxiety** can be provoked by either real or perceived threats, or stressors. These stressors and potential threats are abundant in the veterinary setting. How an individual animal responds to specific events or stressors is unique to each pet, and can change over time with learning history – for better, or for worse.

While the stress of veterinary visits can provoke avoidance, hiding, and defensive aggression, stress and fear can also induce the state of learned helplessness.[2] **Learned helplessness** is a state where an animal (or person) learns that avoidance, escape attempts, or other responses to something unpleasant or threatening are ineffective, and eventually gives up attempts to escape.[2] In pets, this often looks like the pet is "a statue," "frozen," or "stoic." Learned helplessness can mask important findings on physical examination like changes in range of motion, pain in the abdomen, or other findings that rely on patient responses. Conversely, animals who are defensively **aggressive** because of fear may react by vocalizing, snapping, or moving away during examination. This response may be difficult to discern from a pain response, making diagnosis and treatment more challenging. In each of these cases, the animal who is undergoing treatment is suffering emotional distress, and deserves our empathy and respect. Each time the pet visits our office and has a negative experience, the fear will potentially worsen. This learned fear of the veterinary hospital is much easier to prevent than it is to reverse.

Preventing fear in the veterinary office isn't just about stopping the problems associated with fear; it is also about reaping the great benefits of working with patients who are less anxious. Patients who are comfortable and less anxious will allow more complete physical examination; allow better positioning for tests; have more accurate parameters, such as blood pressure, heart rate, temperature, and respirations; have more accurate lab results; and enjoy visits much more. Wouldn't it be wonderful to see patients who are happy to see you? We think so, too!

1.3   Freedom, Wants, and Needs

Dr. Temple Grandin is a world-renown expert in animal behavior and animal welfare. In her book *Animals Make Us Human*, she discusses what are called "The Five Freedoms" in animal care, originally developed by Dr. Roger Brambell in 1965 (Table 1.1).[3] When we cause fear and anxiety in our patients while we are trying to care

Table 1.1 The Five Freedoms.

The Five Freedoms
Freedom from hunger and thirst
Freedom from discomfort
Freedom from pain, injury, or disease
Freedom to express normal behavior
Freedom from fear and distress

Animal welfare is a crucial factor in animal care, and The Five Freedoms were developed by Roger Brambell and popularized by Temple Grandin.

for them, we are infringing on their freedom from environmental discomfort, freedom from anxiety and distress, and freedom to express normal behaviors. One of the first steps in restoring these freedoms is identifying the difference between wants and needs in the veterinary office.

To protect freedom from anxiety for our patients, we recommend setting up guidelines for assessing animals during procedures. We will discuss assessment tools throughout the book, but the first step is understanding when to stop and assess the patient. One guideline for when to stop a procedure involving restraint is to use the 2-2-3 rule. If it requires more than two arms to gently stabilize the patient, if a dog struggles for more than 2 seconds, or if a cat struggles for more than 3 seconds, pause the procedure, assess the patient and the situation, and then make a plan for how to best continue.

Determining when to perform a procedure relies on identifying the difference between wants and needs. **Needs** are urgent, life-saving treatments. *Wants are everything else.* While we may not want to pause or postpone some procedures, pause, retry, or postpone is always an option for wants. By keeping our priorities clear about wants versus needs, we can avoid causing unnecessary harm, and do our very best to keep the stress and fear levels as low as possible for our patients. Keeping fear levels low helps to protect our patients from emotional harm.

1.4 Iatrogenic Behavioral Injury

Iatrogenic means an illness or injury *caused* by medical treatment. Iatrogenic behavioral injury (IBI) is a term to describe mental, emotional, and/or psychological harm caused to patients while we are trying to provide veterinary care. Preventing IBI is one of our responsibilities as veterinary professionals. There are many modalities we can use to prevent IBI, including: recognizing the risks of IBI; using the human pediatric model for most treatments;[4,5] staying up-to-date on medical treatments for fear, anxiety, and stress; and using **low-restraint** and **no-restraint veterinary care**.

The pediatric health care model has changed considerably over the past 20 years. A new emphasis has been placed on the importance of reducing stress for children and parents during medical care. Some techniques used in the pediatric model include explaining procedures to children using words and pictures prior to treatment, bringing comfort items such as a blanket or favorite toy from home, playing music clinically established to have a calming effect, allowing children to sit in a parent's lap and be held or hugged, using distraction techniques, practicing good caregiver continuity, and helping children to cope with pain levels.[5] Medication is given when needed for anxiety or fear, and ongoing research is searching for effective calming methods for children in medical settings. While we can't mirror all of these techniques in veterinary medicine due to the communication barrier between people and pets, we can certainly make use of the concepts to improve patient care.

Veterinary medicine will benefit from the experiences of pediatricians by implementing similar stress-relieving strategies. By explaining a treatment to a child, the doctor or nurse is telling the child what to expect and providing an opportunity for predictability and trust. The veterinary equivalent of this method is "explaining" procedures to pets by using touching and training techniques that help the pet understand what is expected, what to anticipate, and how to **cooperate**. We can allow pets to remain with their owners for many procedures, and coach owners on the best way to assist us. Receptionists can instruct owners to bring a mat, favorite treats or toys, and a hungry patient to each visit. Animal handling staff can become proficient in **distraction techniques** and training methods to reduce animal stress and promote cooperation. We can use medicines and supplements to mitigate fear and stress. For animals who need repeated treatments, we can help them cope by establishing a consent protocol for treatment, instructing the animals how to cooperate, and even sometimes teaching them to look forward to treatments.

If there was a magic wand for making our vision a reality, the authors would make two sweeping changes in veterinary medicine tomorrow: we would implement the use of generous amounts of food treats, and we would allow the owner to be present for most treatments (anesthesia and radiographs excluded for safety and exposure reasons). Working with animals with the owner present allows owners to see precisely what happens between person and pet, and opens the conversation when training and/or medical relief of fear, stress, and anxiety are needed. When the owner is present, veterinary professionals are less likely to resort to "brutacaine" and excessive physical force to accomplish medical care. Furthermore, it helps clients bond with the practice and trust that we have their pet's best interests, both physical and emotional, at heart. Clients can learn how to participate in treatments when appropriate, and how to replicate treatments such as pills, ear medicine, eye medicine, injections, grooming and nail care, and much more at home when needed.

1.5 Introduction to Low- and No-Restraint Animal Care

We will never be able to explain to our animal patients the important protection a vaccine provides, why an antibiotic is needed, what x-rays are for, or any of the other treatments we perform. In veterinary medicine, we have a history of being procedure focused. We tend to make a treatment plan and execute it, with the goal being completion of the procedure. Imagine you're at the dentist for a filling. You like the dentist, and the hygienist is always friendly with you. You sit down in the chair, and without explanation the dentist puts a needle into your mouth to numb the area. You jump slightly at the needle stick; in response, the hygienist holds your arms down against the chair and leans forward, trapping your legs. Your mouth is numb, and the dentist drills

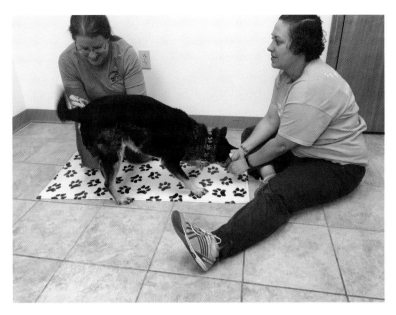

Figure 1.1 Relaxed dog accepting food in the exam room.

while the hygienist holds you down. Your palms are sweaty, and your heart races. You can't stop wondering when this will all be over. What emotions might you experience? Anger? Fear? Anxiety? Even the most easygoing person would probably find this scenario unpleasant. This is an example of **procedure-centered treatment**. What happens the next time you need to visit the dentist? Could the dentist and hygienist have done something differently to encourage you to cooperate? Did they overreact? Perhaps you won't find the dentist's office so pleasant in the future. Perhaps you won't go to the dentist for a few years. This happens with our patients all the time. Restraining even relaxed animals for medical treatments can have similar fallout. Look at the body language of the dog in Figures 1.1 and 1.2. Restraint alone causes a significant change in this dog's body language. Notice the ears pulled back, leaning away, and stiffness the animal shows in response to the restraint without any medical procedures being performed. By focusing more on **patient-centered treatment**, and less on the procedure, we can enhance care and well-being.

Working with animals comes with a risk of injury to the veterinary team and to the animals. We can decrease that risk and increase safety for both the team and our patients by using low- and no-restraint, compassionate care and handling methods. At the time of publishing, the authors have a combined 35 years of experience in full-time veterinary practice. During those 35 years, a grand total of four combined bites have been sustained, and none were serious. Why are we comfortable working with little or no restraint? Because it is effective. These methods can be used safely and effectively with proper education and practice.

Animals use **body language** and body position to communicate with us. Animals can tell us if they are comfortable, **conflicted**, fearful, and anxious, all without any vocalizations or **aggression**. Violence is a biologically costly strategy: it comes with risk of harm for the aggressor. Most animals will exhaust nonviolent means of communication before

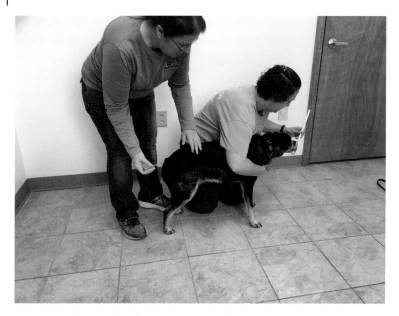

Figure 1.2 The same dog shown in Figure 1.1 when restraint is applied. Note the change in body language.

resorting to defensive aggression.[2] When an animal feels its safety is threatened, the first response most animals use is the flight response: running away from the threat. When we remove the animal's opportunity to leave a threatening situation, we limit their available responses to **freeze** or **fight**. In the veterinary setting, we can become accustomed to ignoring nonviolent communication. When we ignore these important signs, we put ourselves at risk for injury, and the animals at risk for IBI as well.

When we move very close to an animal for manual restraint, we lose the ability to objectively observe the animal's responses and body language. We also send a series of potentially stressful messages to that animal. Research shows that using force when training dogs, such as attempting an **alpha roll** where the dog is forcibly placed on its side or back, can lead to aggression.[6] Placing an animal into **lateral recumbency** or **dorsal recumbency** can similarly provoke aggression. These dogs are not "bad" or "mean"; they are simply responding in a way that is normal for some dogs. When we are working with an animal in sternal recumbency or standing, and we "hug" them to provide restraint, what message does the hug actually send? The word *hug* may hold a positive connotation for humans, but for dogs, hugging is not a natural form of communication. If one dog grasps another around the middle, this is usually displacement, ritualistic conflict behavior, or sexually motivated.[7] It is easy to understand why a hug from a stranger at the veterinary clinic may not seem friendly, and may provoke avoidance or aggression.

There is no such thing as an unprovoked bite in the veterinary hospital, nor a bite without warning. The simple act of bringing an animal into this environment is provocation in itself. It is easy to miss subtle signals in the hospital environment. When we are too close to the animal, we may not see all the signs. Restraint can mask warning signs as well. If the animal is leashed or held, the ability to flee is removed, which masks

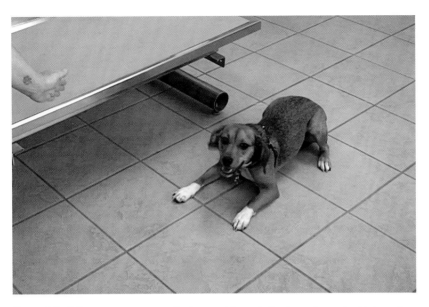

Figure 1.3 Chloe, a young puppy, displays avoidance behaviors when asked to target the technician trainer's hand.

attempts at communication. Removing the option of flight is provocation. Animals who try to get away are warning us about possible future aggression. Animals who freeze, move away, turn to the side, yawn, look away, purse their lips, flatten their ears, vocalize, advance-retreat, snap, and more are all asking us to stop what we are doing. Chloe, the dog in Figure 1.3, is asking the trainer to move away and communicating she is uncomfortable with what she is being asked to do. If we ignore these requests, we run the risk of provoking the animal into self-defense.

Excessive restraint carries physical risks for the veterinary team, including bites and scratches, sprains and strains, and more. There are emotional risks to the veterinary team as well. When our mission, our vocation, is to relieve animal suffering, and we are constantly holding animals down and causing them to experience fear and distress, it can take a toll. Turnover in the veterinary profession is high.[8] Many technicians and veterinarians leave the profession after a short time, while others experience depression and compassion fatigue. Suicide rates among veterinary professionals are staggering.[1] Reducing patient stress may help protect us from these types of emotional harm.

In Video 1.1, the beagle Chloe is expressing anxiety by approaching and retreating. She will come to take food and will make contact with the technician, but immediately backs away between interactions. This backing-away behavior shows the internal conflict this dog is experiencing. She is very anxious, but has not yet escalated to threat displays or defensive aggression. The shepherd mix Max shows a similar pattern of approach-retreat and is conflicted, but he is also vocalizing and lunging, so some would describe him as more aggressive. Both of these patients are doing their best to communicate their discomfort and anxiety by leaving the situation. If we ignore these nonviolent signals, and muzzle and heavily restrain these dogs, we are teaching them that

Table 1.2 Steps for planning treatment.

Pause, assess, prioritize, proceed: Steps for planning treatment
1) Pause treatment: Assess patient and plan.
2) Assess whether the planned treatment is a *want* or a ***need***.
3) Prioritize needs first, then wants.
4) Prioritize wants in order of medical importance.
5) Evaluate the animal's stress level, and the anticipated response to the procedure.
6) Assess if medical therapy for fear, stress, anxiety, pain, etc., is indicated.
7) Make a training or handling plan to help the animal cooperate with as little fear and stress as possible.
8) Proceed with treatment in a fashion that allows the animal to cooperate.

If a patient is showing signs of stress or fear, remember to pause, assess the patient and the plan, prioritize, and proceed while observing the patient closely.

nonviolent communication is ineffective. The dogs will learn the veterinary clinic is a place where subtle signals are ignored, and there is a real risk these dogs will escalate to biting in the future. We don't have to overrestrain these patients. We can work with them and even train them to cooperate in their own health care.

When working with little or no restraint, we will find some animals are unable to allow treatment. They may move away, they may never let us approach them, or they may become defensively aggressive. When an animal can't tolerate treatment, the veterinary team needs to have a plan of action. Table 1.2 provides a quick reference.

1) Pause treatment, and assess the patient and the plan.
2) Assess whether the planned treatment is a want or a need. If the treatment is truly a need, it is life-saving treatment. There are very few situations like this in veterinary practice. A few examples include **GDV** in distress, emergency **dystocia**, animals in severe **shock**, serious traumatic injury with significant active bleeding or respiratory compromise, or the animal is at immediate risk for severe self-harm.
3) Prioritize needs first, then wants.
4) Prioritize wants in order of medical importance.
5) Evaluate the animal's stress level, and the anticipated response to the procedure.
6) Assess if medical therapy for fear, stress, anxiety, pain, or the like is indicated.
7) Make a **training plan** (or handling plan) to help the animal cooperate with as little fear and stress as possible.
8) Proceed with treatment in a fashion that allows the animal to cooperate.

Change is never easy, but it is also often extremely rewarding. This guide will give you the knowledge you need to understand how animals **perceive** their environments, how they communicate, and how they learn. You will learn how to assess a patient, how to tell when to stop a treatment, the steps for making a training plan appropriate for each patient, and assessment of the patient's response to training. Some training plans discussed may take only a few seconds, while others require several visits and compliance from the owner at home. We will also give you the tools you need to help introduce and promote change in clinic culture toward compassionate **cooperative care**. Methods for working with the veterinary team and for approaching topics of concern with clients will be discussed. The animals can be our very best teachers if we allow them, and the rewards associated with a move toward patient-centered practice for both pets and people are worth the effort.

References

1 Skipper, G., and Williams, J. (2012) Failure to acknowledge high suicide risk among veterinarians. *Journal of Veterinary Medical Education.* 39 (1), 79–82.

2 Overall, K. (1997) *Clinical Behavioral Medicine for Small Animals.* St. Louis, MO: Mosby.

3 Grandin, T., and Johnson, C. (2009) *Animals Make Us Human: Creating the Best Life for Animals.* Boston: Houghton Mifflin Harcourt.

4 Kain, Z., *et al.* (2006) Preoperative anxiety, postoperative pain, and behavioral recovery in young children undergoing surgery. *Pediatrics.* 18(2), 651–658.

5 Visintainer, M., and Wolfer, J. (1975) Psychological preparation for surgical pediatric patients: The effect on children's and parents' stress responses and adjustment. *Pediatrics.* 56(2), 187–202.

6 Herron, M., Shofer, F., and Reisner, I. (2009) Survey of the use and outcome of confrontational and non-confrontational training methods in client-owned dogs showing undesired behaviors. *Applied Animal Behaviour Science.* 117(1–2), 47–54.

7 Handelman, B. (2009) *Canine Behavior: A Photo Illustrated Handbook.* Spokane, WA: Direct Book Service.

8 Welborn, L., *et al.* (2013) 2013 U.S. Veterinary Workforce Study: Modeling capacity utilization. In *Report for the American Veterinary Medical Association by The Center for Health Workforce Studies.*

2

Perception and Communication

2.1   Sensation and Perception

Sensation is the way we gather information about the environment around us. Think of sensations as the raw data collected by our sensory organs before the data is translated into meaningful information in the brain. When the sensory data travels to the brain via the nervous system, the brain processes this data into how we think, feel, and react to our environment: our perceptions.[1] One example is hearing. Sound waves enter the ear canal. The waves cause movement within the eardrum and middle ear, and eventually reach the **cochlea**. The waves then encounter the auditory nerve, which transmits the sound signal to the brain. The brain translates this raw sensory data into meaningful information, such as music or speech.

Pets, like people, have a variety of sensory organs. Their senses include vision, hearing, smell, touch, and taste. Animals can also sense **pheromones** using a specialized organ called the **vomeronasal organ (VNO)**, which is part of the **olfactory** system (Figure 2.1). Humans have a VNO as well, but experts disagree about whether humans communicate using pheromones in the same way animals have been confirmed to do. We will discuss sensation and perception in dogs and cats, to help us understand why animals may react in certain ways and make the decisions they do about their environment, particularly the veterinary environment. Dogs and cats have evolved specialized sensation and perception mechanisms.

Sensation and perception are how animals learn about the environment and develop feelings, opinions, and skills. Understanding how animals interact with the sensory environment, and especially noting individual variation, can significantly improve interactions between veterinary professionals and patients.

Vision

Vision contains many separate components, each of which contributes to the total experience of sight.[2] These components include color, acuity (sharpness), brightness (luminosity), **depth perception** or depth sensation, and motion sensitivity. How an animal sees their environment depends upon the anatomy and placement of the eye, and how the brain processes visual data. Humans have a visual field of about 190–240°, with 120° of binocular overlap in the center, where both eyes can access the same visual data, combining the images to assess depth of field.[1] Table 2.1 shows differences between human, dog, and cat vision.

Cooperative Veterinary Care, First Edition. Alicea Howell and Monique Feyrecilde.
© 2018 John Wiley & Sons, Inc. Published 2018 by John Wiley & Sons, Inc.
Companion website: www.wiley.com/go/howell/cooperative

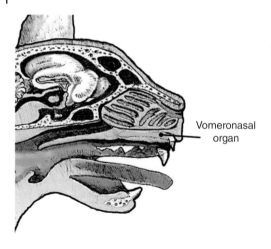

Figure 2.1 The vomeronasal organ location in the domestic cat. This organ is used to detect pheromones.

Vomeronasal
organ

Table 2.1 Sensation: Vision: A summary of human, canine, and feline visual sensations.

Species	Detail acuity	Color	Field of vision	Light receptors
Feline	20/100–20/200	90% fewer receptors than humans	200–295° total 130° binocular	High
Canine	20/80	Bichromatic blue-yellow emphasis	240° total 40–120° binocular	Moderate
Human	20/20	Trichromatic	190–240° total 120° binocular	Low

Canine Vision

How the eyes are placed in the head determines how much overlap there is between what each eye sees. Humans have forward-facing eyes and a 120° field of **binocular vision**, where what the left and right eyes see overlaps to allow depth perception and perspective. Dogs have a field of vision of about 250°, but only 40–120° of **binocular overlap**, depending upon breed and conformation of eye placement. For breeds with the eyes closer together (e.g., Pug), there is greater overlap, resulting in a broader binocular overlap and better depth perception but less peripheral vision. For breeds where the eyes are further apart (e.g. Greyhound), there is less binocular overlap but improved peripheral vision. In general, dogs have broader peripheral vision than humans.[2]

Color is **bichromatic** for dogs. Many pet owners believe dogs see in black and white, but they actually do see in limited color. Based upon the distribution of cones in the dog's eye, they are thought to see the blue and yellow portions of the color spectrum best, with other colors lacking good differentiation.[3] When you see a dog's eyes shining at night, this effect is caused by light reflecting off of the **tapetum lucidum**. The tapetum lucidum and the number of **rods** dogs have given them improved vision in low-light situations. This is an excellent adaptation for hunting, but not helpful for reading. Because of the ratio of rods to nerve fibers, dogs have decreased visual acuity for fine detail, and their vision is more focused on movement and contrast. Their vision is best in close-up situations. We would consider dogs to have 20/80 vision, while humans have 20/20 visual acuity.

In the veterinary setting, if we want to draw a dog's attention to an item like a mat, station, or target, choosing something blue or yellow in color, and placing it on a contrasting background, may help: for example, a yellow or white spoon or a blue plate to deliver treats. Conversely, items we do not wish to draw attention to should be low-contrast and in other colors. When moving ourselves or items around a dog, we can move smoothly and steadily, so as not to trigger a motion-activated overreaction. To draw extra attention to something like a piece of food or a toy, tossing the item so it has added movement, and choosing something of a contrasting color, can improve the dog's awareness of the item. For instance, tossing white cheese bits onto a dark-colored floor, or rolling a dark ball across a white floor, will make these clearer for dogs.

Cat Vision
Cats have a visual field of about 200–295°, with up to 130° of binocular overlap, depending upon the source cited.[4] Their peripheral vision field is similar to that of dogs. Like dogs, cats have less visual acuity for detail, and more focus on movement and contrast. They also have a diminished spectrum for color vision compared with humans. Based on the distribution and variety of cones present in the eye, cats are thought to see few colors. Having only about 10% of the color receptors that are present in the human eye, cats certainly see less differentiation in color than humans do, and based upon research findings, color seems to hold little importance for cats.[3] Like many other animals, cats have a tapetum lucidum that all primates lack, assisting with low-light vision. Even more than dogs, cats excel in low-light situations. Cats would be described as having 20/100 to 20/200 vision acuity if we attempted to classify it in human terms.[4]

As when working with dogs, items that may be alarming to cats should be similar to the background in color, while targets, stations, feeding mats, and toys are best in high contrast. Toys and treats that move around and are high contrast will better draw a cat's attention as well, such as a white spoon or tongue depressor to give food against a darker mat or towel.

Figure 2.2 shows a simulation of the differences in color vision in a common clinic scenario: the exam room. Figure 2.3 demonstrates the comparison between visual fields in humans, dogs, and cats. Figure 2.4 shows a variety of dogs with different eye positions. Consider the impact these eye positions may have on the individual dog's overall field of view, and which areas have best depth perception.

Hearing

Hearing sensitivity or strength is generally defined in terms of what **frequencies** an animal can hear, and how broad the audible frequency range is. The frequencies heard depend upon the anatomy of the ear, which also changes over time. Humans can hear frequencies in the range of 20 Hz–20,000 kHz. Most human speech falls between 1000 and 5000 Hz. As humans age, our ability to hear higher frequencies diminishes. The fine hairs within the ear become stiffer, and the aqueous material in the cochlea thickens. This makes our hearing less acute and sensitive with age. Animals experience similar age-related changes. Like some humans, some animals may be born with changes in hearing or deafness, or may develop these problems prematurely.[5] Table 2.2 shows a hearing comparison between species.

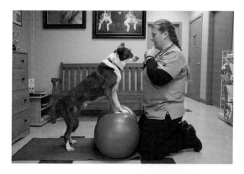 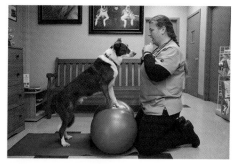

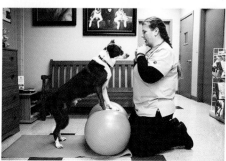

Figure 2.2 Color vision. Color vision based on anatomy of the eye. Top left: Human View. Top right: What we believe dogs see. Bottom: What we think cats see.

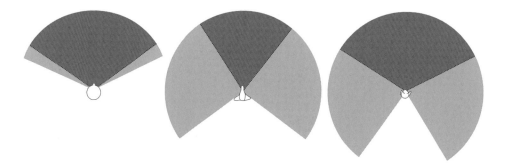

Figure 2.3 Field of vision. From left to right, human, dog, and cat field of vision. The darker shaded area is seen with both eyes (binocular overlap where depth perception is possible), while the lighter shaded areas are peripheral vision fields for each individual eye.

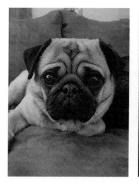 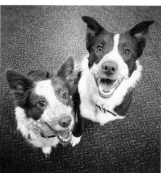 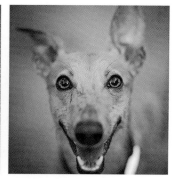

Figure 2.4 Comparison of canine eye set and head shape. Different head shapes and distances between the eyes, as well as where the eye is positioned on the head, will impact the dog's visual field.

Table 2.2 Sensation: Hearing: A summary of human, canine, and feline auditory sensations.

Species	Frequencies	Common sounds at this frequency
Feline	55–79,000 Hz	Piano's low A note: 55 Hz
		Bat echolocation: 50,000–100,000 Hz
Canine	67–45,000 Hz	Lowest cello note: 68 Hz
		Ultrasonic dental scaler: 18,000–45,000 Hz
Human	20–20,000 Hz	Lowest pipe organ note: 20 Hz
		Speech: 1000–5000 Hz

Dog Hearing

Dogs hear a considerably larger frequency range than humans, at 67–45,000 Hz. The frequencies heard best by dogs are around 4000 Hz, which is well within the comfortable range of human hearing.[5] The ultrasonic scalers used in dentistry emit frequencies between 15 and 39,000 Hz. Think about how different your clinic may sound to a dog.

Cat Hearing

Cats hear a considerably larger set of frequencies than even dogs, at 55–79,000 Hz.[5] While they may not be able to hear an elephant's long-range call at 21 Hz, they can hear everything happening inside our hospital. Cats can even hear the lower ranges of bat echolocation, which can span 50,000–100,000 Hz and is completely inaudible to humans.

Think about things in the hospital that may sound different to our patients (Figure 2.5).

Olfaction and Pheromones

Olfaction, or sense of smell, is our ability to sense and perceive odors in the environment. For humans, these smells are detected when molecules of volatile (floating) compounds reach a special area of nerve endings high inside the nose, which is about the size of a

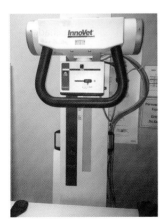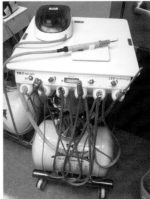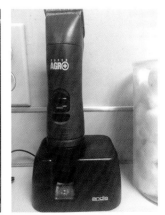

Figure 2.5 Equipment that may sound different or startling to animals in the veterinary clinic. Clippers, ultrasonic dental scalers, and x-ray machinery are a few examples.

postage stamp and contains about 5 million olfactory receptors of 450 different types. Once the odor reaches the olfactory receptor, a chemical signal is sent to the nearby olfactory bulb in the brain. Humans can differentiate about 10,000 different odors, and some of the most noxious odors can be detected in very small quantities, such as one drop in a swimming pool of water! However, most odors are not so easily detected.

Pheromones are detected by the VNO. While humans have a VNO and also secrete pheromones, experts do not agree on whether pheromones are useful for intentional social signaling as an adaptation in humans. There is some evidence suggesting that stress-related pheromones trigger an enhanced startle reflex in humans, which may support subconscious pheromone communication.

Dog Olfaction and Pheromones

Dogs are the experts of olfaction. Their olfactory sensors cover a large part of the surface area of the nasal epithelium. Dogs have a staggering 220 million olfactory receptors in the nose, of about 900 different varieties.[6] Once the odor molecule reaches the receptors within the nose, signals are sent to a comparatively large olfactory bulb, and often the signal must traverse a tiny distance of only one neuron before perception can begin in the brain. Their nostrils can be used to direct and intensify certain odors, and sniffing is done intentionally to obtain olfactory information.

Pheromones are also used extensively by dogs.[6] Pheromones are secreted in association with estrus, pregnancy, lactation, fear, excitement, sexual maturity, health status, and more. When a dog is fearful, it may secrete pheromones associated with fear, and those pheromones can be detected by the next dog who is in that part of the hospital. Pheromone signals can trigger a fear response as the VNO is linked with the **limbic system**. The limbic system is a portion of the brain responsible for emotion, olfaction, long-term memory, and linking emotion with sensation. Synthetic pheromone products such as Adaptil® simulate the pheromone that mother dogs secrete when they are lactating, which is thought to calm the puppies. Using pheromone products in the hospital may help dogs to relax in this environment.

Cat Olfaction and Pheromones

Cats have considerably more olfactory receptors than humans: 150–200 million of at least 500 different varieties.[6] The have a similar percentage of their nasal epithelium containing odor receptors as dogs, and spend a similar amount of time investigating odor in their environments.

Cats also use pheromones extensively, to gather and give information about sexual and reproductive status, age, health, territory, and social cues. Pet owners are most familiar with the use of cheek and chin glands to secrete pheromones during rubbing or bunting, and glands on the paws used during clawing or scratching behaviors. Cats do secrete pheromones associated with emotional status as well, and these messages are left behind in your hospital by each cat who visits for the next feline inhabitant. Synthetic products to mirror pheromones in cats, such as Feliway® (facial pheromone) and Feliway Multicat® (mammary pheromone), can help cats relax in the veterinary setting.[7] When cats (and some other animals) are sensing pheromone information, they may display the *flehmen response*, a characteristic facial expression with the upper lip retracted and mouth slightly open.

Touch

The human body is covered in nerve endings that collect sensory information about touch. Receptors for pressure, contact, vibration, hair movement, heat, cold, pain, position in space, and more are all part of the sense of touch. When a touch receptor encounters a stimulus, a series of signals are sent to the brain for interpretation into a perception of the touch. How dense the nerve endings are in a certain area of the body, and how much of the brain is dedicated to interpreting that data, dictates how "sensitive" that area is to touch. For example, fingertips are very high resolution, packed with 2500 sensors per square centimeter, while the middle of the back may have as few as 500.[8] As you would expect, the parts of the body used for manipulation, exploration, expression, and escape have the highest concentration of touch receptors in both people and animals.

Perception of touch is complex in humans and in animals. For example, if we touch someone who is ticklish under the arm with a feather, the person is likely to react strongly. Touching another subject who is not ticklish in the same way may elicit no response at all, or just a puzzled expression. These two people may have differences in sensation, perception, or both, which shape their responses. Animals are similar in their individuality.

Dog and Cat Touch

The distribution of touch receptors in dogs and cats seems to be similar to that of humans, with the lips, face, feet, and genitals all being quite sensitive. In addition, dogs and cats are special: their vibrissae, or whiskers, give them added sensitivity. These special sensory hairs are located around the face and front feet, and can trigger a strong response when touched or triggered.[9]

When touching dogs and cats, many times the collar can be pulled tight, the paws grabbed, or the lips or face touched when an owner is applying punitive action or when the animal is being restrained or examined in the veterinary hospital. These sensitive areas require special consideration from the veterinary team, understanding how an animal may be startled or frightened by sudden touches. For both dogs and cats, starting touch in a less sensitive area and gliding to a more sensitive area can help the animal's nervous system acclimate to the type of touch required. Figures 2.6 and 2.7 show areas where the sense of touch is more intense shaded in darker colors, whereas regions with lesser density of nerve endings are lighter in color.

Figure 2.6 Sensitivity to touch in dogs. Darker shaded areas are often more sensitive for most patients, while lighter shaded areas are less sensitive.

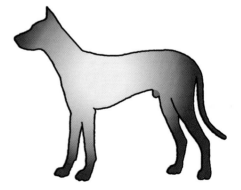

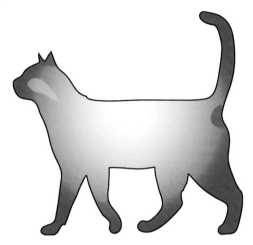

Figure 2.7 Sensitivity to touch in cats. Darker shaded areas are often more sensitive for most patients, while lighter shaded areas are less sensitive.

Taste

Sense of taste is one area in which humans are the winners! While taste and olfaction are closely linked when it comes to determining if a flavor is pleasurable, humans distinguish at least five aspects of taste. Individual taste buds are responsible for detecting sweet, sour, salty, bitter, and savory. Humans have between 4000 and 9000 taste buds of different types located on the tongue, in the oral cavity, and in the nasal cavity. Each taste bud contains 10–50 individual receptors.[8] Taste information travels from these receptors to the brain via the facial nerves.

Dog and Cat Taste

Both dogs and cats have considerably fewer taste buds than humans, with dogs averaging 1700 and cats around 500. Their nerves also seem to process taste considerably differently than human nerves do. Because dogs and cats can't talk, we must again rely on anatomic data and extrapolation to imagine what their sense of taste is probably like.

Studies of the facial nerve, nerve receptors, and brain activity when specific chemicals are offered suggest dogs and cats have the most receptors for sweet and savory. They also have many receptors for bitter, but these receptors are located far back on the tongue where plentiful ingestion or chewing is required. Dogs have more sweet receptors, while cats seem not to respond when the sweet chemical is given. Both cats and dogs have an inhibited response to salts when these chemicals are provided.[10]

When providing foods in the hospital, providing sweet, fatty, and meat-flavored foods generally works best for most dogs and cats. Because olfaction is an important part of taste for pets as well as people, heating foods to increase odor can improve palatability and interest. Food is not the only thing we provide in the veterinary hospital that may trigger a taste response: medicines are important, too. Masking bitter medicines, or encasing them in a capsule so the animal does not encounter the bitter item, can be helpful.

Individual Variations: Nature and Nurture

Animals, like people, will have individual variations that may be **intrinsic** to the animal or learned through experience. It is important to note individual variations, whether they are natural or learned, to best serve every single patient. Some Basset hounds may resist nail trims, because their conformation influences how that touch feels. Himalayans with a reduced visual field may startle more easily when approached from behind. Bloodhounds may detect an odor left behind by a fearful animal more easily than another dog.

When a certain sensation predicts a specific experience, learned aversions can occur. When the odor of ear cleanser predicts a wrestling match followed by touching of a painful infected ear, the smell may become **aversive**. When the smell or taste of a specific cat food predicts nausea in a patient with renal failure, that smell or taste may become aversive in the future. When nail clippers predict touching of the foot and an accidentally painful experience if a quick is cut, nail clippers alone may cause the animal to anticipate a sensation of pain. (Refer to Chapter 3 for more information on classical conditioning.)

2.2   Stress and Fear

Many times when we think of stress or fear, we think of these as bad things. The negative emotions that come to mind when we remember being afraid or being stressed out can make us think stress or fear are always harmful. In reality, stress and fear exist to keep us out of harm's way. The stress response is a combination of instinct, **genetic predisposition**, and learning history. When we are faced with a threat, the sensory organs see, hear, smell, feel, and so on a certain stimulus or group of stimuli. The emotional part of the brain, the **amygdala**, sends a fear message to the hypothalamus, which is like the choreographer of the brain. The **hypothalamus** triggers the sympathetic nervous system to respond, and **adrenaline** is released. The adrenaline release leads to an increase in heart rate, blood pressure, and respiratory rate and capacity, and a release of a bolus of glucose for instantly available energy. In this newly heightened state, we are ready to fight or flee in response to a threat. This response happens extremely rapidly. In humans, the stress response can take less than 0.3 seconds![11] If the perceived threat remains present after the initial stress response, **cortisol** levels are increased and the body remains ready to react in a state of heightened awareness and stress. If the perceived threat is lessened, the **parasympathetic nervous system** moves into action, calming everything down and helping the body to relax.[11]

This stress and fear response helps keep us safe, and it does the same for animals. Without the stress response, we would be unable to respond to immediate threats such as a knife being dropped while cooking, an oncoming car, or a fire alarm. Fear is an important default response, necessary for safety and survival. Especially in the wild, animals benefit from the fear response when it is appropriate. This adaptive trait is helpful, but can become a problem in certain situations.

Puppies and kittens who do not have the benefit of positive **socialization** experiences during youth may never learn to be unafraid in new environments, meeting new people, being exposed to new sounds and surfaces, understanding different kinds of handling, and so much more. These stimuli may trigger the stress response even when the threat is not real. Stress and the fear response are coded in to be the default response when presented with "things" or "experiences" they did not learn were positive and harmless when they were young.[6,7] Furthermore, some animals are genetically predisposed to be more fearful than others. Animals who are predisposed toward a strong fear response and then receive either insufficient or incorrect socialization are at risk for increased

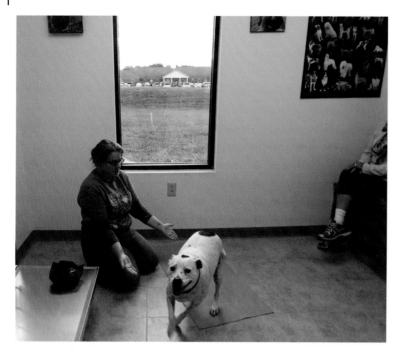

Figure 2.8 Flight response. This dog is fleeing from a fearful stimulus (trainer).

unwanted behaviors at home, and increased handling and veterinary care problems as well.[6] These pets have an intensified feeling of fear in certain situations, which can be maladaptive and harmful to their emotional well-being over time.

When the fear response is triggered, most animals will try to flee (Figure 2.8). Fighting, as mentioned in Chapter 1, is biologically expensive, so most animals will not choose to fight as the first line of defense. If flight is not helpful in alleviating the threat, the animal may feel no choice but to fight. There are a number of ways that the flight response may fail, particularly in the veterinary setting. Sometimes, the animal is in a confined space or wearing a leash. Other times, the animal may have learned that in the past, attempting to flee was not successful and only the fight response stops the threat from becoming worse. In any case, both flight and fight are methods of self-defense that exist to keep animals safe in the presence of a perceived threat.

Preventing fear in the veterinary office is paramount to providing patient-centered care using minimal restraint and intervention. One of the best services that hospitals can provide to prevent fear is positive socialization visits and classes for puppies and kittens, where puppies and kittens have the opportunity to visit the veterinary hospital and learn that the smells, sights, sounds, touches, tastes, and pheromones of the veterinary hospital are nonthreatening and actually predict good things like treats and favorite toys. Qualified team members can lead classes or offer happy visits, so puppies and kittens can practice skills like walking through the clinic, getting treats on the scale, going into the examination room, entering and exiting the cat carrier, and mock physical examinations. Team members can work together with pet owners to set up pleasant expectations about veterinary visits, handling, grooming, and general husbandry. These lessons can transfer in a meaningful way to the client's home relationship with the animal as well, helping to improve the bond between people and pets through good experiences surrounding necessary care for good health and comfort.

2.3   Body Language

Body language is the primary language our animal patients have to communicate with us. Becoming experts in body language can help us better understand our patients, recognize signs of stress and fear early, respond quickly to reduce fear in the veterinary setting, and prevent forming a learned response that can work against us in the future. The purpose of this guide is to help veterinary professionals understand the body language of relaxation as well as mild, moderate, and severe stress using a few key indicators. The guide provided will apply to a vast majority of patients, but individual variation can create animals who are more complicated to categorize. Learning history, differences in sensation or perception, physical illness or compromise, owner perception and communication, and what treatments are attempted will all affect how an individual responds in a given situation.

As we discuss body language, we need to remember that individual breed characteristics influence body language, and contextual cues are crucial to properly interpret body language cues. Some breeds are at a communication disadvantage because of structure. For example, Pugs, Chow chows, Shar pei, Himalayans, and Persians have a difficult time altering their facial expressions because of brachycephaly and excessive facial folds. A Pug with eyes that are bulging and showing the whites can be normal, but this would be abnormal in any German shepherd dog. Basset hounds, Bloodhounds, and Scottish folds will have less ability to communicate using their ears because of their size or shape. Breed differences in normal body posture also exist. Greyhounds holding the ears flat to the head can be normal, but a Corgi doing so is more likely to be fearful. A tail held low and loose between the hocks is normal for a Border collie or a Sheltie, but a low tucked tail for a Labrador or Golden retriever is likely a sign of fear.

Context and the total picture of the animal are very important for accurate interpretation of body language. Both of the authors own dogs who fold their ears back during walks. One is a Jack Russell terrier, and the other is a Border collie. Both dogs are eager to go for walks, and the rest of the body remains loose and relaxed during the walk. The ears alone are not enough information to interpret how the dog is feeling about going for a walk. The entire animal as well as the situation must be considered when making determinations about body language. No animal can be read by his tail alone!

Metacommunication is important, too. Metacommunication is the combination of signals, especially in sequence, to give context to what could be an ambiguous cue. For example, if a dog growls at another dog, growling alone is not helpful information. If the dog first play bowed before growling and moving in a staccato motion away, the growl is likely part of a play invitation sequence. Alternately, a dog who growls after moving away and slinking with a low tail and head is likely showing fear and self-defense behaviors.[9] A cat who crouches, wiggles the rump, and then claws or bites is probably engaging in a play or play-predation sequence. A cat who crouches, leans away, flattens the ears, and then claws or bites is showing fear and self-defense. A growl or bite alone is not useful information: metacommunication helps clarify signals.[9]

In an attempt to make this guide easy to read, we will try to use consistent terminology throughout our discussions about evaluating an animal's emotional state, and choosing appropriate training levels for the state of the animal. There is no single consensus on exactly how to categorize body language and emotional states in animals. Common terms used include ***appeasement***, *conflict*, ***calming signals***, and *aggression*. Experts agree that conflict, appeasement, and calming signals are often prompted by the fear response.[9] This guide will use the following terms to describe and categorize fear and stress in veterinary patients:

- Relaxed or calm
- Mild stress (shows calming signals and/or appeasement behaviors)
- Moderate stress (shows conflict behaviors and/or avoidance)
- Severe stress (shows conflict behaviors, aggression, and/or learned helplessness).

We will describe in detail how to assess stress levels for each canine patient. Table 2.3 provides a summary that may serve as a quick reference guide.

Dog Body Language

Relaxed or Calm, Dog

Overall Impression, Proximity, and Food Acceptance   To read stressed or aggressive body language, we first must know what "calm and relaxed" looks like. When interpreting body language, first observe the whole body. Where is the animal in relation to you? Removing the leash or opening carrier doors so the dog is loose gives the first clue in his comfort level. A relaxed dog will approach, and be willing to remain in close proximity to the team member without retreating rapidly or leaning backward. The relaxed dog will face the team member, and will approach forward or showing the side of the body. He may solicit attention. If he normally likes food treats or toys, he will accept them from the team member. Because the muscles are relaxed, the dog will take food gently or with some excitement, but will not bite hard. A dog with a relaxed body will sometimes lean against you, and will not feel stiff. He may get slightly more still when touched, but immediately soften again. The muscles should feel loose and soft under the skin rather than tense. The haircoat should be flat or in its normal position.

The relaxed dog will usually feel comfortable exploring the room. He is likely interested in investigating his surroundings without being hypervigilant. **Displacement behaviors** (Table 2.4) are absent, and the general impression should make the people in the room feel calm as well.

Training Tip: Normal Vital Signs

Interpreting respiratory rate, pulse, and temperature readings in stressed animals means knowing what normal is.

Canine	Feline
Temperature: 100–102.5 °F	Temperature: 100–102.5 °F
Pulse: Puppies 160–200	Pulse: Kittens 220–260
>6 weeks 60–140	>6 weeks 140–220
Smaller dogs higher	
than larger dogs	Respirations: 20–30 bpm
Respirations: 10–35 bpm	

Table 2.3 Canine body language: Comparison of body language indications connected with different emotional states in dogs.

Emotional state	Proximity	Food acceptance	Body	Face	Tail
Relaxed	Approaches willingly Remains close Solicits attention	Readily accepts food Takes food gently	Front approach Side approach Soft muscles Hair lies flat	Normal pupils Soft eyes Relaxed ears Relaxed lips	Neutral Slightly elevated Wagging softly
Mild stress	Approaches willingly Remains close May lean away when touched	Readily accepts food May take food quickly or roughly during touching May or may not stop eating during procedures	Front approach Side approach Mild tension when touched Relaxed muscles when not touched	Normal pupils Pinched expression Forehead wrinkles Ears slightly pulled to the side or back Looks away when approached Closed mouth Lips relaxed	Neutral Slightly tucked Slightly raised Wagging with mild tension when touched Relaxed wag when owner touches
Moderate stress	May approach for treats Withdraws when food is not offered Leans or moves away when touched Prefers to stay near owner	May take treats Takes treats roughly Retreats after taking treats May refuse treats	Side approach if any Shaking off Panting Lips pulled back Dilated pupils Wide eyes Scratching Other displacement	Pupils dilated Eyes widened Whites of eyes may show Ears flat or pulled back	May wag with tension Tucked
Severe stress	Will not approach Hiding Attempts escape	Refuses most food Rarely accepts high-value food If accepts food, rapidly retreats	Exaggerated movement (fast or slow) Possible piloerection Freeze Vocalize Snap Bite Learned helplessness	Tight muscles Hard eye Dilated pupils Squinting Whites of eyes visible Looks away Stares	If wagging, stiff high wag Tucked tightly

Table 2.4 Displacement behaviors: Examples of behaviors that may communicate anxiety and discomfort when they occur in any context other than the appropriate one listed.

Possible displacement behavior	Appropriate context for this behavior
Shake off	Dog is wet
Yawn	Dog is tired and relaxed
Lick lips	Hungry, food is offered
Scratching	Itchy
Sniffing	Attractive odor present; dog is relaxed
Sneezing	Mechanical or chemical irritant
Grooming	Relaxed dog cleaning himself
Play signals	Relaxed dog inviting play at an appropriate time

Face   The face of a relaxed or calm dog will have relaxed facial muscles. When the face is relaxed, the eye will be neutral. Neutral eyes are not bugged out and appear soft. The whites around the eyes should not show (unless they always do). The pupils should be normal size. The dog should be willing to look at the team member, or at least at their treats. Due to relaxed muscles, ears should lay in a neutral position for that breed. Ears that are typically held upright should be in that position and not turned toward the sides or laying against the back of the head. Some dogs will flatten the ears when petted on the head, but remain relaxed. Floppy ears should seem forward and relaxed as shown in Figure 2.9.

A relaxed mouth is typically held softly closed or open a little. The lips seem soft and loose because the muscles of the face and neck are relaxed. The relaxed dog will not be panting unless he has been exercising or the temperature warrants panting to cool down.

(a)

(b)

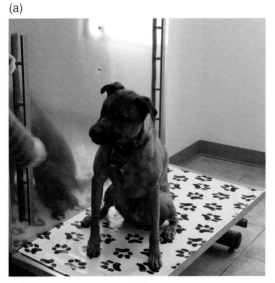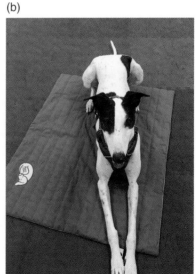

Figure 2.9 (a–b) Two relaxed canine patients.

Tail   As we know from working with so many dogs, not every wagging tail is a happy tail. A relaxed dog has a loose wag that moves the whole butt end of the dog back and forth and practically touches the dog's body on either side. Some breeds will hold the tail loose and low when they are relaxed. Many dogs are missing a tail, and so this piece of information will be absent in those cases.

Relaxed Body: Video 2.1   A Jack Russell terrier holds her ears forward; her body is relaxed. Her eyes are alert but not overly large, her mouth is slightly open and relaxed, and she takes treats with a soft mouth and has quick response to her cues. She will approach the handler and does not back away. The Greyhound has his ears back in a relaxed position for this breed. His body is relaxed and he prances; his eyes are soft, and after taking a treat he is right back to the handler; and his mouth is slightly open and relaxed. The Goldendoodle puppy has a soft wiggly body. Her ears are relaxed and slightly forward, and her tail is loosely wagging. She is taking treats and staying close to the trainer (even though her owner is in the room). The cattle dog is alert and in working mode. She is soft with her mouth and keeps close proximity. Because she is ready for work, her body is not as loose or wiggly, but her ears are up and her face is relaxed; no whites of the eyes are showing. Her movement and focus show she is intense about her work, as she was bred to be. All of these dogs are participating in training nicely and show no signs of anxiety with what they are asked to do.

Excited, No Distress   The excited dog who is not in distress, but is not calm, may be happy to see the team and eager to greet them. The dog may be pulling toward team members, jumping up, whining, barking with a high-pitched voice, and seeking attention. Often these dogs will convert to relaxed and calm body language when their social needs have been met. If the dogs do not become more calm and relaxed after the initial greeting, look for other signs that may indicate mild stress.

Mild Stress, Dog

Dogs experiencing mild stress will generally show stress signals during interaction with the veterinary team and handling events, but will rapidly return to their baseline, more relaxed state when treatments are stopped. These changes can be quick and subtle.

Mildly stressed dogs will often show appeasement or displacement gestures. The body language of appeasement is meant to de-escalate stressful situations and communicate a signal of "no threat," or tolerance but discomfiture. Displacement behaviors seem completely out of context. For example, when the veterinary team member tries to touch the dog, he may return to his owner and offer a known action such as sit or lie down.

Body language such as raising a paw or placing a paw on the owner, leaning on the owner, licking of the chin or face of the veterinary professional, flicking the tongue, lip licking, turning away and sniffing, and yawning are all thought to be de-escalation responses to stress (conflict, appeasement). Several of these gestures, such as licking the face and leaning or pawing at the owner, can be misinterpreted as affection. It is important to consider context: is the animal in a potentially stressful situation? Then the signal is probably a gesture of appeasement. For example, if a dog is turning and sniffing the ground when we attempt to touch him, he is probably stressed. If he turns and sniffs the ground where he found a piece of hot dog a few minutes ago, he could be investigating the environment. Context helps us understand behavior.

Overall Impression, Proximity, and Food Acceptance   A mildly fearful dog will approach willingly and usually look relaxed until you start to handle him. He may or may not explore the room. He will often allow petting, but may lean or walk away sometimes. He will usually approach facing you or with his side to you. He may lean away when petting is attempted. Once handling or procedures begin, stress markers may increase, but in most cases the dog will still accept food and remain nearby to receive it. Mildly fearful dogs will often remain interested in a distraction of delicious treats during handling or a procedure, but the dog will take the food more quickly or slightly more roughly during the procedure. The dog may also stop eating for brief periods during handling, then return to the treats between touches. When touched, the muscles have some tension, and the skin may crawl in an exaggerated **panniculus** response when touched lightly. The haircoat should be lying flat or in its normal position.

Face   Mild stress will cause tension in the facial muscles. The eye may seem pinched, with a small forehead wrinkle. The ears may be pulled to the side or back. If the ears are normally erect, they may point sideways or be laid back. The pupils may be normal size or slightly **dilated**, and the **sclera** (whites of the eyes) are unlikely to be showing. The mildly stressed dog will often look away from the veterinary team member, and frequently look at the owner.

Figure 2.10 shows a dog being touched by the veterinarian, and then being touched by the veterinarian while a treat is offered. The first picture shows taut facial muscles with the ears pulled slightly back. The dog is averting his gaze, avoiding eye contact. The

(a)   (b)

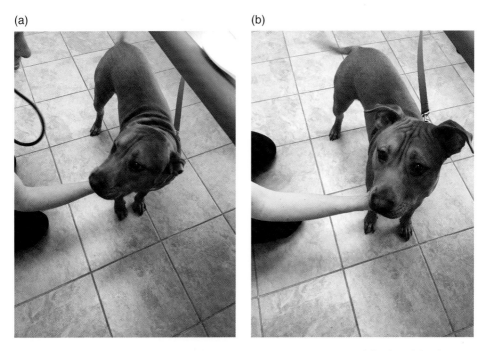

Figure 2.10 (a) The dog is nervous about touching. (b) Touching is paired with food, and the dog is visibly more relaxed.

second picture shows more relaxation in the facial muscles, and the ears are more relaxed. The dog will now make eye contact with the technician as well.

Tail

The tail should be held in a neutral position for the breed. Tension through the muscles of the back and tail causes the tail to be tucked tightly under the dog, or raised somewhat and wagged with mild tension. The tail will change based on what is being done. If the dog is being touched by a veterinary professional, it will probably drop or tuck slightly, and when the touching stops or the owner interacts with the dog, loose wagging or a neutral tail position is expected. Figure 2.11 shows two mildly stressed dogs.

(a)

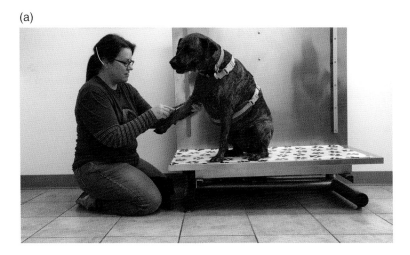

(b)

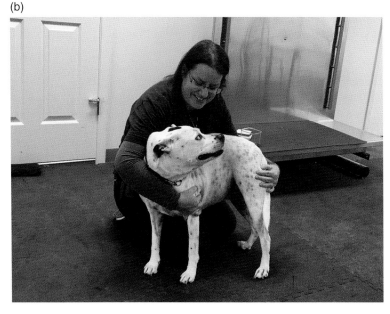

Figure 2.11 (a–b) Two mildly stressed dogs.

Canine Mild Stress: Video 2.3   This first dog in the video, an Australian shepherd, wants to interact with Alicea and is attentive to her food treats. She looks relaxed until she is touched. She has a learned response of showing her teeth during mild or moderate stress, and she does so, but rapidly becomes more calm. She moves her ears forward when she hears a click and receives a treat, but moves her ears back when she is touched. The dog avoids eye contact with Alicea, and when she looks toward the camera it is easy to see her widened eyes. Her rapid changes between mildly stressed and more relaxed show she can return to baseline easily.

The second dog is a brown mixed breed. He is happy to get on the platform and receive clicks and treats, but he is uncomfortable when touched and hugged. The dog is able to tolerate this handling and remains in place for it, but his ear placement and body tension, as well as his averted gaze, show he is experiencing mild stress while he is working and waiting for the click to signal a food reward is coming. While he is experiencing mild stress, he is clearly able to work and make cognitive decisions.

The last dog in the video is the pit bull. She chooses to stay in very close proximity to Alicea and accept treats. Her tail and body are fairly relaxed, but when restraint is performed her tail and body become visibly tense. She has the option to leave the training session, as do all of the dogs in the video, but she chooses to remain in the situation and continue participating. She rapidly returns to baseline relaxation when handling is stopped.

Moderate Stress, Dog

Moderately stressed dogs may show any of the signals of a mildly stressed dog, plus additional displacement, conflict, and avoidance behaviors. Conflict behaviors are usually distance-increasing signals. The dog is asking for more space and for the threat to cease, but is not yet showing signs of overt aggression. When experiencing moderate stress, the dog may be of two minds, not sure how to respond. This indecisiveness is shown through body language. In general, moderately fearful dogs take longer to return to their baseline behavior after stressful experiences, and may not look relaxed while in the hospital at all.

Overall Impression, Proximity, and Food Acceptance   Moderately fearful dogs will often approach the veterinary team member for treats, but will repeatedly withdraw in between taking the food. These dogs may approach quickly (the "snake bite" for treats) or slowly, but they rarely choose to stay near the veterinary team member even when food is obviously available. A dog may stretch his neck way out to reach the food while keeping all his body weight away from the perceived threat so he can escape quickly. This can look like a middle ground between "fight" and "flight." Sometimes the dog has the courage to come closer, and then he may become overwhelmed and need to rapidly retreat. The dog will usually keep an eye on team members rather than turning to the side or away.

Very high-value food can sometimes have a masking effect on moderate stress. It is important to observe how a dog is taking food, and not just whether or not he is eating. To use a human example, we can discuss fear of spiders. If we take a large realistic toy spider and ask a friend who is fearful to touch it, she may refuse entirely, or touch it quickly. If we tape a $50 bill to the spider, she may approach more quickly and stay long enough to take the money, but will then back away again. When we ask our friend, "How do you feel about spiders now?" she will probably respond that spiders are just as scary as ever, but thanks for the $50. Just because she accepted the money, this did not diminish her overall fear.

Moderately stressed dogs may show displacement behaviors. Displaced behavior is out of context for what you would expect given the animal's emotional state. Examples include shaking off when the dog is not wet, yawning when the dog is not tired, panting when not hot, scratching when not itchy, or offering a play bow when not really wanting to play. Each of these signals could be signs of moderate stress.

Face   As stress increases, so will muscle tension. When the muscles of the face become more tense, the eyelids are raised, causing the eyes to widen. The dog will sometimes face away while looking at the threat, or face toward the threat while looking slightly to the side, causing the whites of the eyes to show. Pupils will be dilated, and the animal will often be hypervigilant, frequently looking and listening in different directions and showing heightened awareness for what is going on both in the exam room and outside of it. Dogs may vocalize with a low distance-increasing bark (Video 2.2).

The ears will often be held flat against the head, or pulled far back, showing the tension of the head and neck muscles. The lips can be pulled back in a grimace, tightly closed, or retracted, and the animal may be panting. Dogs who are stress panting generally have wrinkles at the corners of the mouth because the lips are very tense, and the mouth is halfway open with very little of the tongue protruding.

Tail   The tail on a moderately stressed patient may still wag, or it may be tucked or held low. If the tail is wagging, it looks more stiff and less fluid, because the muscles are tense. Figure 2.12 shows two moderately stressed dogs.

Canine Moderate Stress: Video 2.4   Video 2.4 shows five different dogs and how they express moderate levels of stress. The first Beagle is very conflicted about practicing her hand targets with Alicea. She is approaching and withdrawing quickly, panting with the lips pulled back; her eyes are wide, her ears are flat to the head and held back, her tail is tucked under, and she is vocalizing. She also shows some displacement behaviors: play bowing and showing her belly when she does not actually want to play or to be petted.

The next long-haired mixed-breed dog shows the transition between mild and moderate stress. He will eat and approach until Alicea attempts to place her arms around him. Once restrained he stops eating, and avoids the situation by backing away.

The small brown mixed-breed dog is an example of pacing and hypervigilance seen with moderate stress. This dog also does the wet dog shake, lip licking, and appeasement licking the technician's face.

The senior black Labrador retriever is mildly nervous, but escalates to moderate stress when Alicea touches him. He retreats, he stops taking cheese, and his eyes widen. Even though he was initially taking food, his body language shows he is nervous and needs more space and a more cautious approach in order to feel comfortable. His owner is a good example of misattribution, in thinking the cheese has caused the stress response. Many owners are not well versed in dog body language.

Lastly, the Cattle dog mix in the video is recovering from ear infection and the medication process at home was quite stressful. When Alicea touches the ears, the dog shows mild stress. However, when she walks out of the camera's view and picks up the bottle

(a)

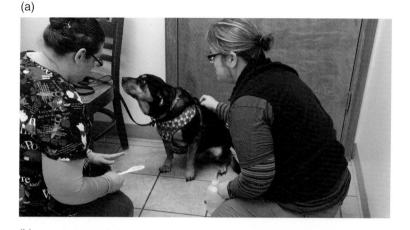

(b)

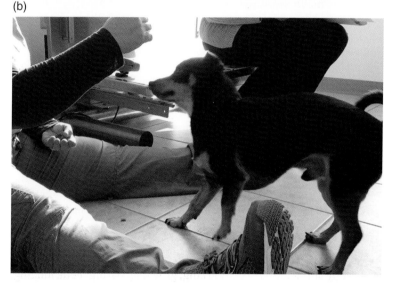

Figure 2.12 (a–b) Two moderately stressed dogs.

of ear medication, the dog's body language completely changes. As soon as he sees the bottle, he stops approaching and immediately turns his focus away, engaging in avoidance and displacement behaviors.

Severe Stress, Dog

Dogs experiencing severe stress are in a state of significant emotional distress. These dogs may show defensive aggression and threatening postures, but this is uncommon. Usually dogs in severe stress due to fear will continue to use hiding and avoidance rather than overt aggression. Dogs in severe distress need relief from their stress prior to attempting training and handling in most cases. A severe state of stress makes it difficult to relax enough to learn new skills and habits. When the emotion of severe fear is linked with the veterinary clinic, animals will find it difficult to cooperate and will often intensify in their reactions over time.

These dogs may show any of the signs described in earlier stress states, combined with those in the upcoming discussion. In addition to body language signals, severely fearful dogs may urinate, defecate, express anal glands, vomit, or even experience vasovagal fainting.

Overall Impression, Proximity, and Food Acceptance   A severely stressed dog will huddle in a corner, hide under a chair or table, or cling close to the owner. The body will be crouched into a ball or drawn in, and they may tuck a front paw under them. The dog will almost never approach the veterinary team member willingly, even when coaxed and offered food. In the rare instance when they do approach, they stay only long enough to grab food and then bolt away. Sometimes these dogs will take food from the owner, or will eat treats that you toss onto the floor, but most often they will not accept food at all.

Once a dog is severely stressed, you will notice everything about his body movements is exaggerated. The dog may move stiffly and slowly, or may frantically scramble at great speed. Some dogs will even enter a state called **learned helplessness**, where they no longer try to escape and seem like a statue. These dogs may appear cooperative, but are in a state of significant distress and suffering.

When approached, a severely fearful dog will become more stiffened or even freeze. This form of freeze is a direct threat, and when backed into a corner or restricted from escaping by a leash, the severely stressed dog may lunge, growl, snap, or bite.

Face   When the muscles of the face are very tight, the eye can look hard. It may be very wide, showing the whites, or squinting. The pupils are usually dilated. The ears will be held tense and tight, usually flat, pulled back, or pulled far forward. Depending on the learning history of this individual, he may avoid eye contact or directly stare at the veterinary team. Often these dogs are hypervigilant, searching for escape routes. If the animal appears exceptionally stoic, he is likely in a state of learned helplessness and experiencing significant distress even if he appears cooperative.

When in severe distress and unable to escape, or having previously learned that escape is not helpful in minimizing the feeling of fear and threat, dogs may defend themselves. Staring directly at the threat, deep barking, growling, baring teeth, lunging, snapping, and biting are all signs of defensive aggression associated with severe stress. It is important to remember that dogs rarely "try to bite." If a dog snaps near someone without biting, in most cases this is a threat that was intended to be an **inhibited bite** rather than a missed attempt at making contact.

Tail   The tail on a severely stressed animal may wag in a staff-like shortened wag but will often be tucked up under the dog. Sometimes the tail is so tightly tucked that the tip touches the abdomen. Figure 2.13 shows two severely stressed dogs.

Canine Severe Stress: Video 2.5   Video 2.5 shows severe stress in five different dogs.

Cricket Boone, the Beagle mix, is sick and must have blood collected this day. She is very nervous and will not accept the peanut butter until after we are done with the procedure. She shows avoidance behavior with her head only and does not move her body away, which is amazing for her stress level. She has a learning history of coming in for happy visits, so this may have helped. Although she is frozen, each step of the process

(a)

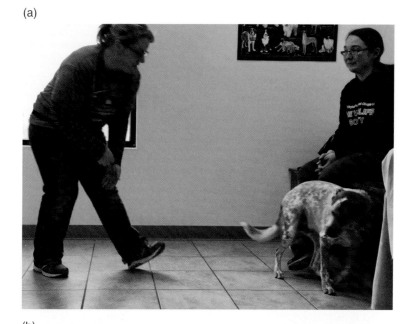

(b)

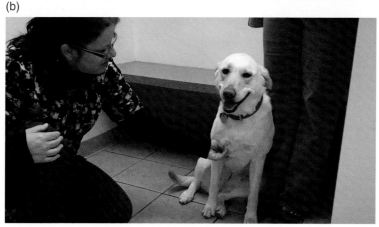

Figure 2.13 (a–b) Two severely stressed dogs.

causes her stress level to escalate. She freezes when touched, vocalizes when alcohol is placed, and vocalizes with the needle stick. She is able to take food after the blood draw is completed. While waiting for blood results, she is able to play with a stuffed Kong toy.

Next is Coco, the Australian shepherd from a previous video, meeting a new team member. As soon as the stranger enters, the dog's eyes widen, she moves slowly, then she freezes. She vocalizes using an alarm bark.

Chris, the Hound mix shown next, is an example of learned helplessness secondary to severe stress. She shows a complete lack of active behaviors and just looks the other way. She appears eerily stoic, which is often confused with the animal being relaxed and cooperative. This dog is very distressed, even though she is motionless.

Max, the Shepherd mix, is showing body language much like the first Beagle, but he is older with a longer learning history, so he is also barking and growling. His nervous approach-and-retreat behavior, avoidance of proximity, looking away a few times, and almost play-bow-like stance confirm this is fear behavior from a very conflicted dog. Notice he will take the cheese even with all the stress, but the manner in which he takes the food shows how fearful he is.

Lastly, Sunshine the yellow Labrador retriever shows clear fear behavior. Her face is so tight that her eyes look sleepy. She tries to avoid Alicea, but the owner pushes her back down. She is panting, and her ears are pulled flat to her head; her tail is tense and motionless. She lip-licks and nose-licks, and she finally stops trying to communicate and enters learned helplessness.

Cat Body Language

Cats communicate through body language, olfaction and pheromones, and vocalizations. Olfactory communication is very important in cats. Each cat has his or her own smell, and cats in colonies have a communal scent, which is why it is important to methodically introduce a new cat into the household or re-introduce a cat that has been at your facility.[12] As with dogs, there is considerable individual variation among cats as well. Some cats are very social depending on their socialization history and genetics, while others are not social at all. Cats who are more social are often more comfortable in unfamiliar environments like the veterinary hospital, but these social cats also feel more confident showing how they feel, and when they are fearful this is often misunderstood as resistance or fractious behavior. As with dogs, signals from cats and the stress level of a cat can change rapidly. Watching for subtle changes and continuously monitoring the patient's state of mind by observing body language cues are the best ways to assess stress levels in cats.

As with dogs, we have divided the language of cats into four categories:

- Relaxed or calm
- Mild stress (mild conflict behaviors and/or avoidance)
- Moderate stress (conflict behaviors and/or avoidance)
- Severe stress (shows conflict behaviors, aggression, and/or learned helplessness).

We present a detailed evaluation guide here, as well as a quick reference summary in Table 2.5.

Relaxed or Calm, Cat
Overall Impression, Proximity, and Food or Tactile Acceptance　A relaxed cat will come out of her carrier on her own at a moderate pace. She will not look rushed or panicked when exiting the carrier. The relaxed cat should slowly emerge while taking in the environment with her nose. She may approach and solicit attention by bumping the veterinary professional with cheek rubs or the top of her head. She will not retreat when you reach out to pet her, and will allow touching without retreating. When stroked, her muscles feel soft and relaxed to the touch. The relaxed or alert cat will often be sprawled out on the exam table or floor, lying on a hip with the legs relaxed and extended. She will also feel comfortable walking around the room with a horizontal back. She will rub on items in the environment, such as chairs or the corners of the exam table, and calmly

Table 2.5 Feline body language: Comparison of different signals associated with the emotional state of cats.

Emotional state	Proximity	Food or tactile acceptance	Body	Face	Tail
Relaxed	Exits carrier willingly Approaches team members Rubs Solicits attention Remains close	Will accept food May show interest in food but not eat Continues eating during handling May show interest in toys May show desire for tactile	Front approach Side approach Soft muscles Sprawls on floor or table Rolls Haircoat is flat	Normal slit pupils Soft eyes Relaxed ears Whiskers neutral	Relaxed Held soft and high Possible curled tip Away from body if lying down
Mild stress	Exits carrier willingly Approaches tentatively Slinky walk Retreats intermittently	May accept food May show interest but not eat Stops eating during handling May stop accepting tactile during handling	Side approach Mild muscle tension Sits or lies down with paws folded	Tense expression Shortened neck Squinting or slightly wide eyes Mild pupil dilation Whiskers neutral or pulled forward	Held low when walking Gently tucked around body when lying down
Moderate stress	Rarely exits carrier Retreats when approached Does not approach vet team Allows owner to approach and touch	Refuses food Refuses tactile	Looks away Hypervigilant Tense muscles Twitch or flinch when touched Mild piloerection	Moderate pupil dilation Widened eyes Ears to the side or back	Down Tucked Tip may twitch
Severe stress	Will not exit carrier Curls up small crouched in back of carrier Avoids approaches Avoids touch	Refuses food Refuses tactile	Tense muscles May crouch May arch back Piloerection Strike with paws Vocalization Bite Learned Helplessness	Dilated pupils Neck tense, short neck Wide eyes Flattened ears	Tucked tightly Stiff swishing Twitching Piloerection

investigate. Her haircoat should be lying flat and soft. She may try to initiate play by chasing or rolling. Relaxed cats will often accept food, and after several visits even begin to anticipate treats in the veterinary clinic. Many relaxed cats will eat food during handling procedures, or will just stop eating briefly for a few seconds during handling. Cats who prefer tactile rewards will accept cheek, chin, and/or head stroking before, during, and after handling and procedures.

Face   Relaxed cats will have relaxed facial muscles just like relaxed dogs. Cats lying on the table may roll onto one side, or rest their heads on the table. The eyes may be softly squinting or open, but don't appear wide. Pupils should be slit, and a normal size for the ambient light in the room. Ears should be held in the normal position of front facing and erect, or slightly to the side especially when touched. Whiskers will be held neutral to forward. Vocalization may occur in the form of friendly or inquisitive meowing or purring, but other vocalizations are uncommon in the relaxed cat.

Tail   Relaxed cats have relaxed tails. If the cat is laying down, the tail will be held straight out on the surface or loosely wrapped in toward the cat. When standing, the tail will be held loosely down but not twitching. As a relaxed cat approaches and solicits attention, the tail will often be raised straight up, but feel soft to the touch, with or without a curled tip. Figure 2.14 shows two relaxed cats.

Relaxed Body Language – Feline Video 2.6   Video 2.6 shows cats with relaxed body language in the veterinary setting. Notice the first juvenile cat is relaxed enough to play with the fishing pole toy, cheek rub, and accept tactile reinforcement from Alicea. The cat's body is loose, ears and whiskers are in neutral position, and eyes are normal in size and dilation. The second cat is eating while being examined by the veterinarian. She allows touch and never moves away even though she is unrestrained and free to do so. The third cat is eager to follow Alicea to her medication station. She is alert, with her tail up and a loose body, and follows Alicea's finger target up onto the training platform.

(a)

(b)

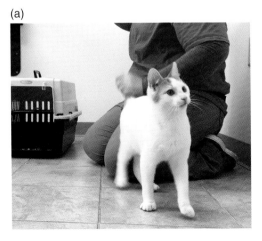

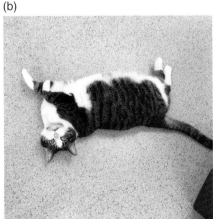

Figure 2.14 (a–b) Two relaxed cats.

Mild Stress, Cat

Overall Impression, Proximity, and Food or Tactile Acceptance   A cat experiencing mild stress may emerge from the carrier right away, or may take several minutes to come out during the history. She will move slowly or with caution, exploring and often looking for a place to hide. While she is walking around the room, the mildly stressed cat may look slinky, with the rear end held low in a crouched walk. The cat may tentatively solicit attention by bumping or rubbing, but she generally retreats after a few seconds of contact. When stroked, her muscles feel slightly tense, and her skin may crawl slightly when she is petted. Her haircoat should be smooth and flat. The mildly stressed cat will often sit, or lie down on her belly with her paws folded. She will not sprawl on her side like the relaxed cat. The cat experiencing mild stress may accept high-value food, but will almost always completely stop eating during handling, and will only sometimes return to the baseline level of food acceptance when handling is completed. Cats who prefer tactile may accept some cheek, chin, and/or head stroking before and after touching or handling, but during touching or handling they may move away for brief periods and then return.

Face   The mildly stressed cat will have tense muscles in her head and neck, causing a tense facial expression. She will not move her head around much, and may even crouch with the neck shortened and the head retracted. Her eyes may be squinting or slightly widened, with mildly dilated pupils. Her ears may be soft and forward, but will more likely be held slightly to the side or back. Whiskers will be in a neutral to forward position; and if the cat is vocalizing, they may meow or what Kessler describes as a *plaintive meow.*[13] Some moderately stressed cats will purr.

Tail   The mildly stressed cat will hold the tail low when she is walking, and will gently tuck it around her body when lying down, often with the tail tip twitching. Figure 2.15 shows two mildly stressed cats.

Feline Mild Stress: Video 2.7   Video 2.7 shows two mildly stressed cats. The first cat is relaxed until it is time for her vaccination. She moves away from the veterinarian, and curls to make herself smaller. She tries to hide against the veterinarian's arm and avoids touch. The second cat takes time to come out of her carrier. Her ears are held slightly back, and she is hypervigilant, checking her surroundings repeatedly. (She is wet because her owner gave her a bath immediately prior to the visit.)

Moderate Stress, Cat

Overall Impression, Proximity, and Food or Tactile Acceptance   The moderately stressed cat will rarely exit the carrier on her own. If she does, she will be tentative in her movement. She may initially move to come out, but then retreat to the back of the carrier again. When the carrier is disassembled and the top removed, often she will sit in the carrier bottom and look away from the veterinary professional. Sometimes, she will "hide in plain sight," nestling into her bed or the corner of the carrier, but still looking around periodically. She may also hide by pressing against or into a team member. Most moderately stressed cats will allow the owner to pet and touch them. She will not solicit petting or touching from the veterinary team, and will move away when handling is

(a)

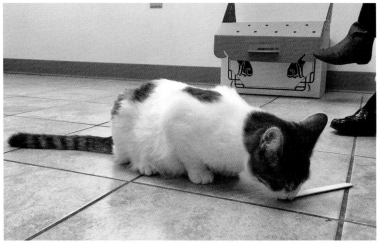

(b)

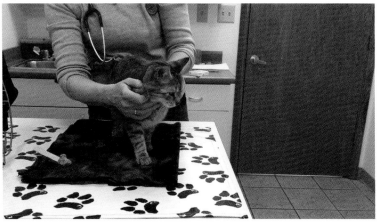

Figure 2.15 (a–b) Two mildly stressed cats.

attempted. If she is moving around the room, she generally darts from hiding place to hiding place, or slinks along the walls, avoiding people. When touched, she may flinch. She is often hypervigilant, noticing noises and movements and responding to them in an exaggerated way. Her coat may show mild piloerection. She will not accept food.

Face　The facial muscles will be tense, so the eyes will appear wider. Her pupils will be mildly to moderately dilated, and she will alternate between looking away from the veterinary professionals and looking at them. She will hold her ears to the side or back, but they will not be completely flat.

Tail　Her tail may be held down or tucked under her body, and if the cat is aroused it will twitch some. Figure 2.16 shows two moderately stressed cats.

(a)

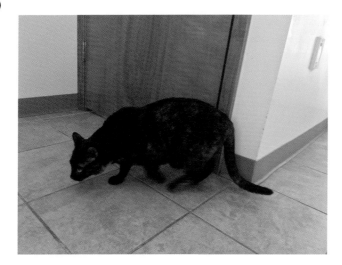

(b)

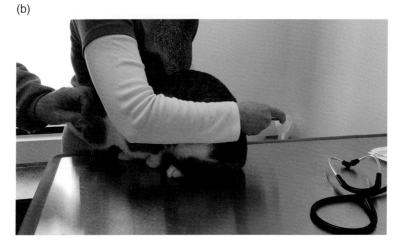

Figure 2.16 (a–b) Two moderately stressed cats.

Feline Moderate Stress: Video 2.8   Video 2.8 shows two cats experiencing moderate stress. Notice the first cat is scanning the room looking for a retreat or hiding spot. Her ears are held slightly back, and she is moving away from Alicea with cautious motion. The second cat is relaxed and eating until Alicea tries to apply some eye medication. The cat switches to moderate stress markers, repeatedly trying to back away, licking her lips, and swishing her tail.

Severe Stress, Cat
Overall Impression, Proximity, and Food or Tactile Acceptance   The severely stressed cat will generally show either some level of defensive aggression, or total learned helplessness. She typically won't come out of her carrier by choice, so the carrier will need to be disassembled around her. When she is in the carrier, or if she is in the exam room outside of the carrier, she will make her body small and tuck her paws and tail close to

the body. If moving around the room, the severely stressed cat will be crouched low to the ground, or possibly stand with the back arched and haircoat standing on end ("Halloween cat"). When the veterinary team attempts to touch the cat, she may rapidly try to escape, hiss, growl, yowl, or strike with a front paw. She may also roll slightly to use her front or hind paws to kick out.

When in severe distress and unable to escape, or having previously learned escape is not helpful in minimizing the feeling of fear and threat, cats may defend themselves. Staring directly at the threat; vocalizing, including meowing, hissing, yowling, and growling; showing the teeth with an open mouth; air biting; and biting are all signs of defensive aggression associated with severe stress. Like dogs, cats rarely "try" to bite. If a cat bites near someone or bites them softly, this is a warning associated with extreme stress.

In some cases, cats will also enter a state of learned helplessness. This seems most common in shy and fearful cats, and shy feral cats. Cats in learned helplessness look like they are trying to be invisible. A severely stressed cat in this state will seem like a statue, and will not respond in the expected way to a given stimulus. She will generally hide her head and look away, close her eyes, or stare off blankly into space. When touched, she will not react or will have a minimal or slow-motion reaction, and she generally does not notice things like vaccinations. Cats in learned helplessness are experiencing severe stress, even though they may look cooperative on the surface.

Face   The head will often be lower than the body, and if the cat is hugging a wall or in a carrier she will turn her face away from you. She will open her eyes wide, with dilated pupils. The ears will be flattened to the side or fully back on the head. Due to the tenseness in the cat, the whiskers will be pulled back; and the cat may hiss, growl, or yowl, although often these cats are quiet.

Tail   The severely stressed cat will hold her tail close to the body and may tuck it under the abdomen, similar to a stressed dog. The tail may swish stiffly, twitch, or remain stiffly still. Piloerection is common on the tail, making it look bigger, especially if the cat is arched. Figure 2.17 shows two severely stressed cats.

(a)   (b)

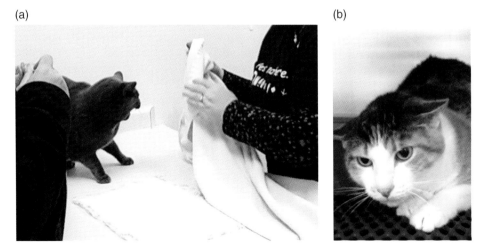

Figure 2.17   (a–b) Two severely stressed cats.

Feline Severe Stress: Video 2.9 Video 2.9 shows three examples of severe stress. The first cat's ears are held flat against her head. Her pupils are dilated, she licks her lips, and her front foot is ready for swatting in preparation for self-defense. The second cat's ears are held back but not completely flat. His pupils are dilated, his whiskers are forward, he hisses when the cage is opened, and he is ready to strike with a front paw. The third cat moves away from Alicea, demonstrating avoidance. She shows tail swishing once wrapped in a towel. During the injection, you can see the cat tense her muscles, back up, hiss, flatten her ears, and crouch.

2.4 Causes of Stress in the Veterinary Setting

Overview

This lengthy discussion of interpreting body language in our animal patients serves to help us identify their stress levels and stay safe, and improves their experiences in the veterinary hospital. Avoiding all stress in the veterinary setting is virtually impossible, but a great deal of stress can be mitigated through understanding, planning, and developing a great knowledge of learning and training. If we understand the causes of stress in our patients, and how the signs of stress can change over time, we can respond rapidly and with the necessary skills to decrease stress where possible, and treat it when needed.

Pain

Pain is a major source of stress in the veterinary hospital. Whether the pain is acute or chronic, even the most well-behaved patients can be stressed, including severe stress and defensive aggression, if they are in pain. Pain can be associated with injuries, infections, osteoarthritis, chronic illness, cancer treatments, gastrointestinal discomfort, pancreatitis, dermatologic disease, and glaucoma, just to name a few. Patients who are aggressive because they are painful due to an injury are learning that the veterinary hospital is a place where pain happens, and the people in the clinic cause painful experiences. This experience can color her future opinion about the environment and people she encounters in the clinic, because they become associated with the painful injury and treatments. After a painful event, it is common to have patients who were once quite comfortable for veterinary care refuse to enter the building, or show extreme fear on subsequent visits.

We encourage liberal use of analgesics and sedatives for painful patients. A good pain management program can go a long way toward keeping team members and patients safer. If a patient is going to require repeated rechecks such as wound dressings, cast changes, **radiographs**, or lab work, it is a good idea to consider the use of **anxiolytic** medications along with the pain management protocol. Patients who struggle due to fear as well as pain are at a higher risk of physical injury in addition to the emotional consequences we have just discussed. Whenever a patient is seen for an acute painful trauma, it is a good idea once the animal has recovered to schedule some happy visits where no treatments are performed. This can help restore trust between the veterinary professionals and the patient, and improve emotional feelings about the environment.

Examination and Treatments

The stress of being touched, having to interact with strangers, and entering an unfamiliar environment can have a considerable impact on patients. Many pet owners can't restrain their animals, brush them, clean their ears or teeth, or clip their toenails even in the comfortable and familiar environment of the home. Now the patient is in the veterinary hospital and needs many of these potentially scary types of handling, and they are being done by a stranger as well. Imagine that a patient, who is showing the mild signs of stress discussed earlier in this chapter, is in the hospital for an examination. The patient looks away, turns away, is panting even though she is not hot, and shows displacement behaviors like sniffing the ground when she is approached. Because the patient is not actively trying to escape, and is not behaving aggressively, veterinary professionals tend to soldier on, providing the physical examination. Imagine what might be going through this dog's mind: "I'm really uncomfortable and I keep telling you, but you're still touching me," or, "This is a really scary place! Please don't come any closer!" and yet we continue touching the animal. These animals are doing their best to communicate their mild and moderate fear to us, but we persist in our examination because we are not forced to stop by their behavior. Consider the learning history this animal is accumulating: nonviolent methods do nothing to prevent this discomfort and scary event. What is the motivation for the animal to continue using nonviolent communication with us in the future? Very little.

It is important to consider that the very things we are doing to try to help our patients, examinations and treatments, provoke a great deal of fear for some animals. Responding with respect to the signals an animal gives us about their discomfort is the first step in building trust and being able to provide more treatments with less stress over the lifetime of the animal.

Trigger Stacking

We have all had that day. We get a speeding ticket on the way to work, the doctor is running 40 minutes behind on appointments, the phone is ringing off the hook, a dog in the kennels can't stop barking, a coworker accidentally stole our lunch out of the fridge and ate it, and then you get a paper cut on your finger while unpacking boxes. That paper cut might cause quite an emotional outburst! Tears, swear words, or storming off might all happen, as a result of a tiny paper cut. But wait: is it really about the paper cut? No, it is about *trigger stacking*. The paper cut was the proverbial "straw that broke the camel's back." **Trigger stacking** is the process where many small stressors increase the emotional sensitivity of a learner (human or animal) over time, and when the learner goes over threshold for emotional resilience, even a small stressor can provoke a large, out-of-context response.

Trigger stacking happens in the veterinary hospital all the time. If a cat is brought into the hospital and experiences this tall stack of triggers, his emotional resiliency may be used up:

- Capture and stuffing into the carrier.
- Carrier slides around on the seat of the car while driving.
- A dog sniffs and barks at the cat in the lobby.
- The owner dumps the cat out of the carrier onto the exam table.

- The owner's cell phone goes off during the history, causing a loud noise.
- A dog in the kennels is barking and can be heard from the examination room.
- The technician takes the cat's temperature and leaves the room.

After all this, when the veterinarian attempts to **auscult** the cat by sliding a hand under the chest to listen, the cat may lash out. The defensively aggressive display is probably not related exclusively to the auscultation, but rather is the culmination of all of the stressors erupting in an exaggerated response. Figure 2.18 illustrates an example of trigger stacking.

An awareness of trigger stacking helps us keep patients calmer during visits. By minimizing all possible environmental stressors, we can help preserve the pet's emotional resilience to cope with an examination and treatments. Furthermore, by using animal-friendly techniques during the examination and treatments, we can continue to expand the animal's emotional resilience. Awareness of animal body language will help us remain in touch with possible trigger stacking, and stay sensitive to an accumulation of stress that may harm the patient's ability to cooperate today and in the future.

Video 2.10 shows a veterinary visit from the cat's point of view. Consider all the possible triggers this cat experiences, and how he might respond when it is time for his checkup and vaccinations.

Learning History

Multiple factors come together to build the learning history of the animal. Each visit, each experience, each event the animal endures in the veterinary setting will contribute to the animal's overall body of learning. Every interaction we have with an animal is a training session, whether the training occurs by intent or by accident. We may be setting up the environment for success by making the clinic inviting: this is passive training. We may be taking a purposeful role to teach our patients we are nonthreatening and can be fun: this is active training. Sadly, veterinary professionals are fantastic at accidentally using both kinds of training to teach our patients to dislike and fear us. On social media, at continuing education conferences, and anywhere else a group of veteri-

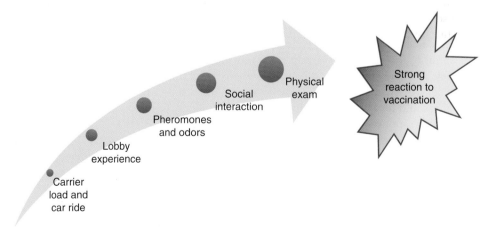

Figure 2.18 Trigger stacking occurs when stressors build one after another, until the patient has a strong response to what may otherwise be a mildly provoking stimulus.

Figure 2.19 By providing more pleasant than unpleasant experiences in the environment, we can help tip the learner's emotional scales in favor of an overall pleasant emotional response.

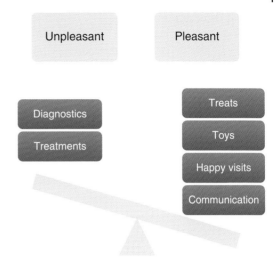

nary professionals gathers, people tend to start swapping war stories. Why do people do this? Are they proud of surviving a harrowing event? Does it show a level of bravery to return to work after being harmed by an animal? Is it a sign of willingness to put the safety of the animal above the safety of the human, allowing ourselves to be injured? We aren't sure why battle scars seem to hold so much value for veterinary professionals, but we are confident the veterinary team are not the only ones with emotional and/or physical scars from these incidents.

For each white ghost of a healed scratch drawn across a hand, every dented thumbnail, every game of connect-the-dots of puncture wound scars, there is an animal who experienced that event as well. Every suture, every antibiotic pill, every ripped pair of scrubs or extra load of wash due to a patient releasing bladder or bowels is a sign of a pet who was terribly distressed while in our care. Our hope is we can begin to learn from our battle scars that there is a better way. Listening to our patients when they talk to us about stress and fear, developing new skills to use when we work together with the animals we love, and learning to set the stage for success for both people and pets will serve us all so much better.

By teaching animals that more good can come from the veterinary hospital than bad, we can help improve their opinions about the setting and the events that happen here. Ken Ramirez talks about the balance between pleasant and unpleasant in the learning environment. The goal is to make sure the pleasant side of the scale holds far more material than the unpleasant side (Figure 2.19).[14] Veterinary care will never be entirely without holding still, being touched and manipulated, needles, clippers, pills, and more. Certainly, if we make an effort to balance the scales in our favor with treats, toys, play, desired touching, and good communication, we can improve the overall experience of our patients and build a more favorable learning history over time.

Steps for Success

To successfully implement the strategies contained in this book, veterinary professionals will need to pay attention to our patients. We will need to assess and reassess pets as we work with them each day, each hour, each moment. We will try to set up the environment and our protocols to improve the patient experience, and we will write down our triumphs. Where? In the medical record! Dedicate a part of the medical record to the patient's likes, dislikes, emotional status, and handling history. These notes should be success based, not warnings. Avoid labels like "fractious," "bites," or "dangerous." Instead, select useful information to help the people who come after trying to handle the same patient. Examples include: "will allow saphenous blood draw with peanut butter spoon," "allowed full exam after trazodone administered at home, remind owner to give trazodone," or "has muzzle from home, loves goldfish crackers." These messages still provide us with the information to approach an animal with caution (as we should with every animal), but serve the additional purpose of reminding us to approach the animal with compassion and a plan for success.

References

1 Goldstein, E.B., and Brockmole, J. (2016) *Sensation and Perception*, 10th ed. Chicago: Wadsworth.

2 Miller, P., and Murphy, C. (1995) Vision in dogs. *Journal of the American Veterinary Medical Association.* 207 (12), 1623–1634.

3 Jacob, G.H. (1983) Colour vision in animals. *Endeavour.* 7, 137–140.

4 Peters, A. (2002) *The Cat Primary Visual Cortex*. Atlanta, GA: Elsevier.

5 Strain, G. (2011) *Deafness in Dogs and Cats*. London: CABI.

6 Overall, K. (2013) *Manual of Clinical Behavioral Medicine for Dogs and Cats*. St. Louis, MO: Mosby.

7 Shaw, K., and Martin, D. (2015) *Canine and Feline Behavior for Veterinary Technicians and Nurses*. Ames, IA: John Wiley & Sons.

8 Norback, C., *et al.* (2005) *The Human Nervous System*. New York: Humana Press.

9 Landsberg, G., *et al.* (2013) *Behavior Problems of the Dog and Cat*, 3rd ed. Edinburgh: Saunders.

10 Serpell, J. (1995) *The Domestic Dog: Its Evolution, Behavior, and Interactions with People*. Cambridge: Cambridge University Press.

11 Gray, J. (1971) *The Psychology of Fear and Stress*. New York: McGraw-Hill.

12 Crowell-Davis, S., *et al.* (2004) Social organization in the cat: A modern understanding. *Journal of Feline Medicine and Surgery.* 6 (1), 19–28. http://journals.sagepub.com/doi/abs/10.1016/j.jfms.2003.09.013

13 Kessler, M., and Turner, D. (1997) Stress and adaptation of cats (*Felis silvestrus catus*) housed singly, in pairs, and in groups in boarding catteries. *Animal Welfare.* 6, 243–254.

14 Ramirez, K. (2011) *Problem solving: Full course on training*. Chicago: Shedd Aquarium Society.

3

Learning, Conditioning, and Training

Every interaction with our patients is a learning experience for them, which means it is a training opportunity for us. Understanding the science of how conditioning and learning happen allows us the best opportunity to assure great experiences for our patients. Selecting appropriate methods begins with agreeing to "Do No Harm," and expanding protecting wellness to include emotional and psychological wellness, as already discussed in this book. Understanding the how and agreeing on the why also let us select an appropriate what: what methods to use for our training. Dr. Susan Friedman provides a model for selecting methods that are most effective at achieving teaching, least intrusive to the learner, and lowest risk for the learner and the trainer.

Dr. Susan Friedman's "Hierarchy of Behavior-Change Procedures" (Figure 3.1) provides a roadmap for making the most ethical choices when training.[1] Along the road, the map shows a series of turns and speedbumps. Each turn represents a training method that can be employed. The first turns available have the least potential for harmful side effects, while later turns could have more concerning possible outcomes. Each speedbump indicates the need to slow down, and proceed with caution only after completely assessing the road ahead. To address a change in behavior, the first stops along the roadmap are to assure the animal's basic needs for wellness and nutrition are being met. Next come **antecedent arrangements**, **positive reinforcement**, **differential reinforcement of an alternate or incompatible behavior**, **extinction** and **negative reinforcement**, and finally **positive punishment**. This is a lot of jargon packed into a few sentences. By the end of this chapter, you will be able to define each of these terms and many more, and apply them to common scenarios in a practical and scientifically sound way.

3.1 Classical Conditioning

Classical conditioning, also known as Pavlovian or respondent conditioning, was defined by Ivan Pavlov while doing research on salivation and digestion in the early 1900s. Pavlov found that his dogs would begin salivating at the sight of the experimenter or the sound of the bell long before any food was presented. While the experiment on digestion encountered a roadblock, Pavlov instead successfully defined a type of learning that was reflexive. He discovered that when a neutral stimulus is presented before an unconditioned stimulus, after many pairings the neutral stimulus will become

Cooperative Veterinary Care, First Edition. Alicea Howell and Monique Feyrecilde.
© 2018 John Wiley & Sons, Inc. Published 2018 by John Wiley & Sons, Inc.
Companion website: www.wiley.com/go/howell/cooperative

Hierarchy of behavior-change procedures

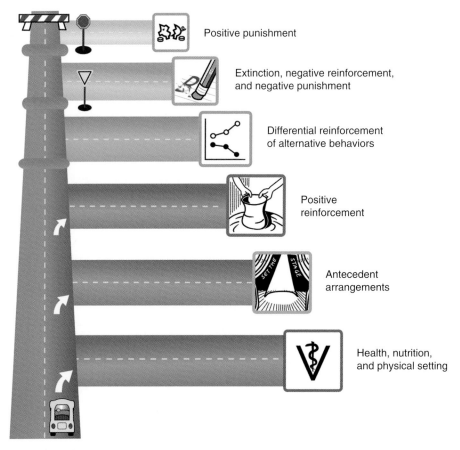

Positive punishment

Extinction, negative reinforcement, and negative punishment

Differential reinforcement of alternative behaviors

Positive reinforcement

Antecedent arrangements

Health, nutrition, and physical setting

Figure 3.1 Roadmap of interventions. Dr. Susan Friedman's guideline for least aversive to most aversive procedures to change the behavior of animals.

a conditioned stimulus causing a conditioned response (Figure 3.2). These conditioned responses are reflexes, secretions, and emotions. The responses are not under the learners' control: responses happen *to* them, and they don't choose to respond.[2] For example, an owner opens the drawer and picks up the nail trimmers, catches the dog, and wrestles to cut the toenails, causing an emotional response of stress and fear. This process is repeated a few times, and when the owner picks up the nail trimmers in the future, this causes the dog to experience the emotional response of stress and fear, even if no nail trimming is attempted.

Classical conditioning is a powerful tool that can work for us or against us in veterinary medicine. Classical conditioning is the science of associations where one thing predicts another. When Pavlov rang his neutral bell, it predicted meat powder. Meat powder causes salivation in the dog. When this predictive relationship was repeated for enough trials, the sound of the bell alone was enough to prompt

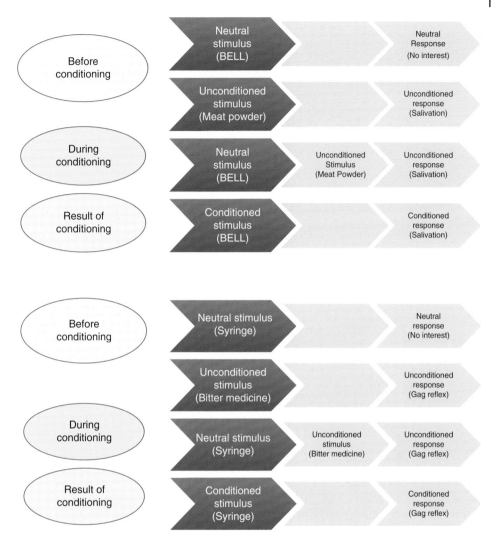

Figure 3.2 Classical conditioning in the veterinary hospital. The neutral stimulus becomes a conditioned stimulus through the conditioning process, resulting in a conditioned response. The first diagram shows Pavlov's familiar experiment on salivation in dogs. The second diagram uses the example of giving a cat bitter medicine.

the response of salivation, without the meat powder being present at all. Pavlov's dogs would hear a bell, and then salivate. What does a bunch of drooling dogs have to do with cooperative behavior? Plenty! Classical conditioning is the reason why cats hate carriers, dogs hate white coats, and the bottle of ear cleanser sends Fido running. The sounds of treat bags, can openers, the owner's voice, and the clicker are all great examples of classical conditioning. Classical conditioning is an extremely useful tool for preventing the development of fearful responses to veterinary handling or procedures (Figure 3.3).

(a)

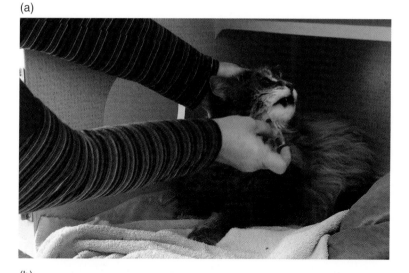

(b)

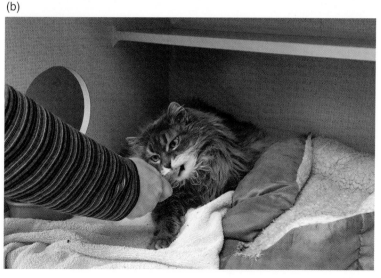

Figure 3.3 (a) Classically conditioned gag response. (b) Classically counterconditioned pleasant response.

Video 3.1: Feline Classically Conditioned Response

The cat here is displaying a classically conditioned gag reflex. This patient has received medications from a syringe that were bitter and made her gag. The medications were the unconditioned stimulus, and the gagging is the unconditioned response. The sight of a syringe is a neutral stimulus until it is paired with the medication inside. Now seeing any syringe, even an empty one or one containing water, makes the cat gag before medication is placed in the mouth. The syringe has become the conditioned stimulus, and the gagging is now the conditioned response. Due to classical conditioning, she gags and spits, even though she has just been given water from a clean syringe. This response is not under the cat's control.

3.2   Operant Conditioning

Operant conditioning, also known as instrumental conditioning, is based on E.L. Thorndyke's Law of Effect (1898) and B.F. Skinner's three-term contingency.[3] Unlike classical conditioning, which deals in unconscious responses, operant conditioning focuses on voluntary behavior where the animal makes choices and these choices lead to **consequences**. Trial-and-error learning is a good way to describe operant conditioning. The learner performs behaviors, and depending upon the consequences, the learner will make future decisions about certain behaviors based upon how those trials and errors were perceived. Figure 3.4 breaks down the quadrants of operant conditioning as they generally apply to animal training.

In most cases, there are two potential categories of consequences for any behavior: **reinforcement** or **punishment**. Reinforcement is anything that increases the future frequency, intensity, or duration of the behavior. Punishment is anything that decreases the future frequency, intensity, or duration of the behavior.[3,5,6] Consequences drive future behavior, whether the consequence is reinforcement or punishment. The trainer will be able to tell whether consequences were reinforcing or punishing by observing the frequency, intensity, and duration of the behavior throughout the training period.

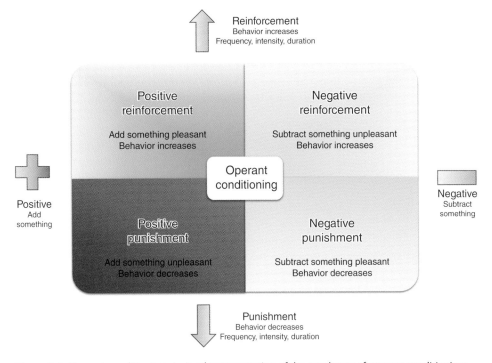

Figure 3.4   Operant conditioning. A visual representation of the quadrants of operant conditioning: positive reinforcement, negative reinforcement, positive punishment, negative punishment. Positive reinforcement is shown in green because it has the smallest probability of unpleasant side effects for the learner. Negative reinforcement and negative punishment are yellow because they present a medium risk. Positive punishment is shown in red because it presents the highest risk of unwanted side effects for the learner.

Technically, we do not know in the moment if we are providing a reinforcing consequence. The animal's behavior over time is the only way to determine if a consequence was truly reinforcing or punishing. There are two types each of reinforcement and punishment: positive and negative. With respect to operant conditioning, *positive* means adding something to the situation, and *negative* means removing something from the situation. These combinations result in positive reinforcement, negative reinforcement, negative punishment, and positive punishment.

Positive Reinforcement

Remember: in operant conditioning, positive and negative do not mean good and bad. Instead, think of them as mathematical terms. Positive means adding something to a situation, and reinforcement means the behavior strengthens over time. So positive reinforcement is the process through which a behavior gets stronger because of what was added to the situation.[3,5,6] Positive reinforcement training has been found to be extremely effective, and it is very popular with trainers around the world for all species.[6] This method instructs the learner exactly what the desired behavior is, and allows the trainer and the learner to have a relationship based on predictability, pleasant interactions, and trust.

The process of positive reinforcement training relies on the learner performing different behaviors, and the trainer delivering consequences. When the consequence is positive reinforcement, the trainer delivers something they think the animal desires and enjoys. The animal performs a desired behavior, and the trainer immediately delivers a probable reinforcer such as a treat, a toy, praise, attention, or touch. How will the trainer tell if what she delivers is truly reinforcing? Simply wait to see if the animal repeats that same behavior in the future more frequently, with greater intensity, or with longer duration.

Example: Teaching a Puppy to Sit

The trainer will wait for the puppy to sit, which is a natural behavior most puppies do fairly regularly. As soon as the puppy sits, the trainer offers a piece of tasty food. If this is reinforcing, the puppy will sit again. If the food is not reinforcing enough, he may try other behaviors, become distracted, or disengage. Environment and individual variation have a great deal to do with motivation, or how reinforcing a learner may find a particular reward.

Example: Teaching a Kitten to Come When Called

The trainer will watch for opportunities when the kitten is moving toward the trainer, and produce a fishing pole toy to play for a few seconds when the kitten arrives at the trainer's feet, then stop playing and move away. If the toy play was reinforcing, the kitten will probably come to the trainer again, and the trainer can then engage in play once more.

Negative Reinforcement

Negative reinforcement is the removal of something to increase the likelihood the behavior will happen again.[3,5,6] Remember: negative doesn't mean bad, it means subtract. Negative reinforcement can present ethical dilemmas, because we are sometimes removing something the animal will work to avoid. This means we have potentially applied something aversive, or put the animal in a situation where aversion is occurring. In general, when we work with animals, we want to choose the least invasive, minimally aversive, and maximally comfortable method for each individual animal. Negative reinforcement should be used with great care for this reason.

Example: Fastening a Safety Belt

When the driver gets into the vehicle and starts the car, a harsh beeping noise occurs. As the driver fastens his seatbelt, the annoying beep stops. In the future, the driver rapidly fastens his seatbelt (increase in belt-buckling behavior) and the beep is removed (negative), so negative reinforcement has occurred for the behavior of seat belt fastening. This example is relatively benign because the learner is able to comprehend the entire interaction in advance, choose to perform the desired behavior, and avoid the beeping entirely, and the aversive stimulus is a nonthreatening beep.

Example: Teaching an Animal to Stand Still When Restrained

The trainer can apply pressure around the animal's body while it is struggling. As soon as the struggling ceases, pressure is removed. The trainer removed something (pressure), and the animal stands quietly more in the future (increase in behavior), so negative reinforcement occurred for the behavior of standing still. The problem with this technique is that the trainer held the animal while he struggled. Struggling is likely a sign of stress or fear in this animal, and this method could damage the trust between the trainer and the learner because the feeling of fear or stress is very unpleasant. Negative reinforcement requires the learner to want to avoid something and have it removed. *We must question the appropriateness of causing intentional avoidance, and be aware of possible fallout from doing so.*

Struggling or resistance to handling should follow the 2-2-3 rule. If more than two gentle arms are required to stabilize the patient, if a cat struggles for more than two seconds, or a dog struggles for more than three seconds, pause the procedure and make a new plan. A different technique is required, and negative reinforcement is contraindicated.

A Word on Punishment

Punishment by its very definition is effective in changing behavior, but it carries disadvantages. Punishment can cause stress and conflict, which both reduce learning efficiency.[6] Punishment also inhibits behaviors, which can mask normal behavior and mask changes in behavior. For example, physically holding a dog in lateral recumbency may cause him to learn to stop struggling, but it also may simply inhibit struggling because he is unable to express his normal behavior since he is restrained. Punishment-based training methods have also been correlated with increased fear and aggression in the learner.[4] Fear may be of the trainer, equipment used, the environment, or a combination of these. Aggression may be displayed toward the trainer or redirected onto other people, animals, or objects. Increased fear and aggression can put patients, clients, and team members at risk. If behavior can be modified using reinforcement, it is our ethical responsibility to choose reinforcement first.

Negative Punishment

Negative punishment describes removing or subtracting a stimulus to weaken a behavior over time.[3,5,6] In general, negative punishment removes something the learner wants, so through trial and error the learner realizes his behavior does not achieve any pleasing result. By removing something a learner wants, we can communicate with a learner that a behavior is ineffective at obtaining rewards. However, this method does not teach the learner what the desired behavior is, and can result in confusion, frustration, and diminished trust between the learner and the trainer. Because the technique involves punishment, it deals entirely in reducing behaviors, but does not increase desired behaviors. While cessation of some behaviors is necessary, this method should be used with caution, as with all forms of punishment.

Example: Teaching a Puppy to Stop Jumping Up   Most puppies jump because they are seeking attention. If the puppy jumps and the trainer steps away, looking away and removing all attention, the puppy may learn that the behavior of jumping up results in removal of attention. If the behavior of jumping up gets weaker with time, this form of training is negative (remove attention) punishment (decreased jumping).

While this punishment is not aversive to the puppy, it also does not teach him the proper way to greet by sitting politely. As mentioned, one problem with punishment is it doesn't teach the learner the desired behavior. As an alternative to punishment, using positive reinforcement by teaching the puppy to sit when a person approaches achieves the same result as forbidding jumping, with the added benefit of the puppy performing the correct behavior. The fastest route to right behavior is to define and then teach the desired behavior (Video 3.2).

Positive Punishment

Punishment, like reinforcement, can be positive and negative. Positive punishment is the addition of something to decrease the likelihood the behavior will happen again.[3,5,6] Positive punishment should be reserved for the last resort if it is used at all in training, and it is not appropriate for veterinary and husbandry training. The use of punishment, and particularly positive punishment, can be challenging. Difficulties include the fact that the trainer needs to be able to directly link the punishment with the behavior in the learner's mind. It is common for the learner to associate the aversive stimulus with the trainer, the environment, or an object rather than the behavior the learner was performing. In addition, the aversive stimulus must be sufficiently unpleasant that the behavior stops, and must occur as a consequence every single time the behavior occurs.[3]

Example: Stopping Drivers from Speeding   Many drivers exceed the speed limit on a regular basis. If you are this driver, you engage in the undesirable behavior of speeding nearly every day. Occasionally you will get pulled over by a policeman, and given a warning or a ticket. Say this happens once every year or less. No one likes getting a speeding ticket, so why do people still speed even after having to pay a ticket? Because the speeding ticket does not meet the criteria for punishment. If it did, the speeding behavior would decrease! Instead, the driver is being intermittently reinforced for the behavior of scanning for police officers and slowing down when they are visible. For speeding tickets to be effective, they would need to be delivered immediately anytime the driver exceeds the speed limit, and the dollar amount would need to be high enough that it was truly aversive.

Example: Stopping Drivers from Running Red Lights Red light cameras are popping up in neighborhoods all over the United States. Drivers know that if they run the red light, they will be mailed a ticket every time they choose to do the behavior. Because the aversive stimulus of the ticket happens every single time the behavior occurs, the punishment should be effective in reducing the number of red lights a driver chooses to run. However, not every light has a camera. The true behavior being changed is a decrease in running red lights where the driver knows there is a camera, not the behavior of running any red light. Some drivers may even choose an alternate route to avoid the lights with the cameras. Punishment is complex to apply properly in a fashion that truly and permanently diminishes behavior.

The Role of Marker-Based Training

Marker-based training, commonly called **clicker training**, is a positive reinforcement strategy used by trainers to improve communication between the trainer and the learner.[6] The clicker is a small plastic and metal device used to make a "click" sound (Figure 3.5). The click is an event marker or **conditioned reinforcer**. The animal experiences repeated pairings of clicking and then treating, and through classical conditioning the animal learns the click predicts a treat. In many cases, the click itself will cause a visible pleasure response in the animal once it is truly a conditioned reinforcer. However, a click is also a promise. A click will always be followed by a **primary reinforcer**. If the pairing of the click with a primary reinforcer is stopped, the value and importance of the click will diminish over time.

The purpose of the click is to mark the precise instant the learner has performed the desired behavior. With human learners, this system is called TAGteach™. You will notice most of the videos show the use of the clicker. We prefer to use the clicker while introducing a new behavior whenever possible, even placing it under our feet when necessary. You will also note the use of a verbal marker in the videos for established behaviors or when the use of a clicker is impractical.

(a)   (b)

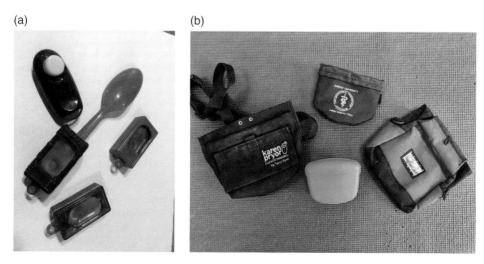

Figure 3.5 (a–b) Clickers are a tool often used in marker-based training. A treat pouch is a convenient way to store food rewards during training.

Using marker-based training allows the trainer to communicate clearly and precisely with the learner. Rewards need to occur within 2 seconds of the correct behavior for the learner to properly associate the reward and successful reinforcement to occur, with a shorter interval such as 0.5 seconds being most effective.[5] The clicker allows this degree of precision. After we "charge" the clicker (or marker word, light, etc., as appropriate for the learner), we can use the click to tell the animal precisely when the right behavior occurred, and use the click as a bridge meaning, "That's right! A treat is coming soon!" The bridge helps span the time gap between the behavior and delivery of the primary reinforcer. Often, we will be training behaviors where the animal can't eat at the same time he is performing the behavior. For example, nose targeting is impossible to perform at the same time a treat is being delivered: when the animal opens its mouth to receive the treat, the nose target behavior will be interrupted. We need a way to communicate with the animal that the right behavior has occurred, and a reward is on the way. The click, or marker, is how we can communicate this information, and can even be used when the animal is far away from the trainer or the treats.

Some research suggests that a click or whistle speeds up training when contrasted against a verbal marker or no marker. Other research asserts that a verbal marker and a click are equally effective if the trainer is very proficient. The authors' experiences suggest that a click is a very expedient bridge that is easy to teach to the learner and to pet owners, so we will use clicker training as our examples a majority of the time.

Marker-Based Training: Mechanics Matter

Our companion animals are very attuned to our body language. Sometimes this awareness is for better, and sometimes for worse. If the trainer moves around a lot or talks to the animal frequently during training, the animal can become confused while trying to figure out what all the movements and words mean. If the trainer stands still like a statue or a robot, many animals will find this suspicious and unnatural, and be reluctant to participate. When initiating a training session, the trainer should be standing in a relaxed neutral posture, with a pleasant facial expression.

Training Tip: Treat Type Matters!

Select tiny treats the animal thinks are delicious. The treats need to be easy to eat quickly (Figure 3.6).

Animals quickly make associations between stimuli or actions, especially the ones that predict food or another primary reinforcer. For example, many dogs come running at the sound of the crinkle of a plastic food wrapper, because that sound predicts food. Many dogs will also give the trainer extra attention when she reaches into her treat pouch or pocket, because that action predicts food delivery. For marker-based training, it is very important that the animal learns the click or marker is what predicts food, not another movement or hand-in-pocket. Choosing a home base position while training is a useful way to prevent misunderstandings. Keeping hands at home base is an easy way to remember to keep the marker as the most important piece of information. Examples of home base include hands behind the back resting in the small of the back, hands at

(a)

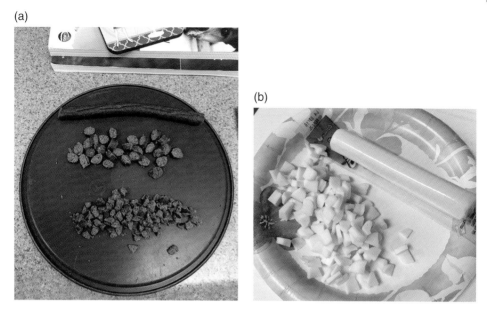

(b)

Figure 3.6 (a–b) Cutting treats into tiny pieces helps make the food easy to eat quickly and controls caloric intake from training sessions.

the sides, or hands folded in front over the waistband. Trainers need to be careful not to rest hands on the treat bag or pocket while at home base. When clicking, keep the clicker hand still, then deliver a treat following the click.

The mechanics should look like: observe desired behavior → click while at home base → reach for and deliver treat → return to home base. Figure 3.7 illustrates this progression.

Marker-Based Training: Capturing

There are two common marking methods trainers use to get behavior from an animal: **capturing** and **shaping**.[6] When capturing, we mark a behavior the animal is already doing in order to strengthen the behavior.[6] The completed behavior is something the animal already offers. For example, puppies are born with the ability to sit. Getting puppies to sit on cue is easy using capturing. Video 3.3 shows Cookie, a ten-week-old Australian cattle dog mix, learning to sit for treats in the exam room. Alicea stands with a treat bag and a clicker handy, and when the puppy sits to scratch herself she clicks and treats. Next, the puppy sat in a more regular pose (just to see Alicea better) and earned another click. Soon the puppy remains in a seated position, so Alicea starts clicking and tossing or delivering the treat, and the puppy gets up to get it. By delivering the treat away from the puppy, Alicea provides the chance to start the sit again, earning another click and treat. Rewarding in this fashion allows numerous repetitions in a short period of time.

Capturing can be used in the exam room for those patients who already do a nice job holding still. For example, the dog chooses to hold still while a nail is clipped. We can click/treat for the stillness and cooperation to capture it, and then proceed to the next

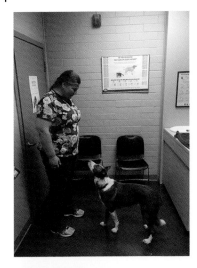
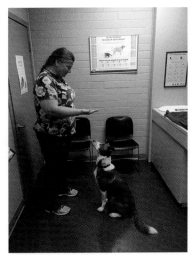
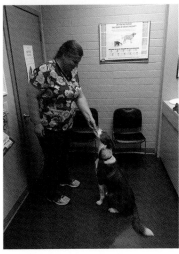
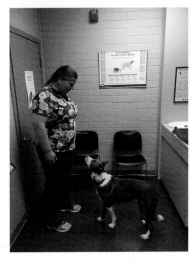

Figure 3.7 Mechanics of marking and delivering rewards. Begin in the "home base" training position (top left). Cue or wait for the learner to offer the behavior. Click when the desired behavior occurs. Deliver a reward, then return to "home base" for the next repetition.

toenail. If we take the time to capture the stillness for each nail and give a treat afterward, the likelihood for calm nail trims in future visits will increase. The temptation is high to just keep going when an animal is cooperating, but it doesn't teach the animal what the desired behavior is. If we ignore desired behavior, it will eventually fade away. Capturing is a great way to maintain or increase desired behaviors the animal is already offering. Furthermore, if we proceed while the animal is calm, and only pull out treats when the animal is wiggling or less cooperative, we are actually ignoring the calm behavior and reinforcing the wiggling behavior. It's important to recognize when animals are already doing something right, so the trainer can make the most of existing desired behaviors.

Marker-Based Training: Shaping

Shaping is different from capturing because we build a complex behavior that is novel: the learner doesn't already perform this behavior. Shaping means breaking down the goal behavior into many tiny pieces, steps, or **approximations**. Pure shaping allows the learner to experiment in the environment, and the trainer will click when a step toward the goal occurs. The trainer will not be prompting, luring, or cuing during shaping sessions.[6] One analogy is the "Hot and Cold" game many of us played as children. The person who is the guesser tries to find or do a "secret" thing. The guide tells the learner they are "getting warmer" or "hot" when they are on the right track, and that they are "cold" when they are wrong. Clicks during shaping are like telling the animal he is "getting warmer," In shaping, we ignore the "cold" part of the game, and only focus on successful approximations of the goal behavior. As animals learn the shaping game, they begin to understand that a few seconds without a click means they aren't on the right track and need to try something else. For shaping to be successful, the trainer needs to have keen observation and good timing. Late clicks, missed opportunities for clicks, and accidental clicks can lengthen the training process considerably. However, errors made using marker-based positive reinforcement methods will not be harmful to the animal or to the relationship between trainer and animal, unlike errors made using punishment.

Shaping allows training of simple and complex behaviors, and it allows the learner to discover the desired behavior through communication with the trainer. When working with an animal on a shaping project, it is important to remember that the learning track is not always linear. While the Hot and Cold game analogy assumes the learner makes constant progress toward the goal behavior, sometimes shaping is more like putting together a puzzle with many pieces. If the goal behavior is the entire picture in the puzzle, each puzzle piece may be an approximation. The shaping process allows the animal to obtain all the puzzle pieces, and learn how the pieces come together to comprise the goal behavior. To become proficient at shaping, a trainer must learn how to maintain the learner's motivation level, and develop a good communication style with the learner. We must watch for communication about what the animal understands, and what the animal has not yet grasped. Shaping relies on a good balance between rate of reinforcement and adjusting criteria. If the **rate of reinforcement** is too low (too much time between treats) or the criteria for reinforcement are too high (task too difficult to earn a treat), the animal may choose not to participate because the task is unclear or too difficult. If the rate of reinforcement is very high, the criteria may remain the same too long, and the animal may begin to think that the goal behavior has already been achieved. The rate of reinforcement must be kept high enough to maintain the animal's interest, but not so high that there is no desire on the part of the animal to try new behaviors or improve through the approximations to attain a more complicated goal behavior. When both the trainer and the animal understand the shaping process, achieving goal behaviors can be amazingly quick.

The key to using any training method successfully is defining what the desired behavior is, and building that behavior by design. Rather than asking ourselves, "How do I stop the animal from jumping up?" the question should be, "How do I teach the animal to sit to greet people?" Instead of, "How can I hold the animal down to get it to stop struggling?" we should ask, "How can I teach the animal to stand still and volunteer for this procedure?"

Video 3.4 shows a Boxer puppy Simba's first experience with shaping. She has never been introduced to the shaping game before, and has only been exposed to the clicker during one other session. This is a novice dog with an advanced trainer. If you are new at clicker training, you should shorten your sessions instead of training for ten minutes like the video shows. You will notice when Alicea first sets the cone down, the dog sniffs it; Alicea clicks to capture the behavior, but because she is a new learner, the puppy does not understand and walks away. That's when the shaping begins. Alicea clicks for any attention toward the cone, whether it's a brief glance, sniff, or walking toward it. Alicea stays consistent with her criterion, and the puppy figures out she should touch the base of the cone. Once the puppy understands the desired behavior involves the cone, Alicea waits for Simba to experiment with touching other parts of the cone, then clicks her for touching the tip, which is the goal behavior.

Video 3.5 shows the use of shaping for Mama Kitty to move onto a scale. The same rules apply to shaping with this cat. She is Hillview's clinic cat and is familiar with clicker training and the shaping process. A cat who is new to training may need more time and more repetitions to understand the behavior. This video is a great example of how quickly an animal can learn a new behavior once they have learned the training game. Alicea first clicks for looking at the scale, then stepping toward the scale gets a click and treat. Mama Kitty then rubs her chin on the scale and gets a click and treat; after that, she keeps rubbing (happy kitty). Alicea waits, and Mama Kitty lifts her foot; Alicea clicks. Mama Kitty then decides the best path onto the scale and puts two paws on, earning a click and treat. After two repetitions, she places all four paws on the scale. This skill took seven clicks for a total of seven calories.

3.3 Habituation, Sensitization, Desensitization, Counterconditioning, and More

Habituation

Habituation is a type of non-associative learning, and is largely a passive process. It is an adaptation where we learn to filter out unimportant information in the environment and stop responding to it. The learner may notice the stimulus at first and respond, but will stop responding with repeated exposures.[6] During habituation, the animal learns the stimulus has no consequences (good or bad), so no response is necessary. In habituation, the stimulus is always presented at the same level, with repeated exposures over time. For example, when you need to turn on your heat in the winter, your dog probably notices the first few times the furnace roars to life. However, this response quickly fades and the dog stops noticing. People who live near the airport may notice the sound of planes flying overhead for a few weeks, but then stop noticing this sound. Similarly, someone who lives near the railroad track may stop noticing passing trains with repeated consistent exposures. Consistent repetition is a key of habituation. If someone who lives near the airport goes on vacation in the quiet wilderness for a few weeks, the sound of planes will be noticed again when they return home. If the stimulus is too intense, for example a car alarm, habituation may never occur. It is very unlikely for a learner to habituate to a very intense stimulus.

Flooding

Flooding is exposing the learner to a feared stimulus at a high level of intensity until they stop reacting.[6] This type of exposure requires the animal not be able to move away from the stimulus until the visible fear response has completely subsided. Most animals display a severe fearful response during flooding, and then will gradually become exhausted and stop responding. The animal will generally try to escape, show visible signs of significant distress, and may become aggressive while trying to avoid the feared stimulus. Some animals will enter a state of learned helplessness, where they are still fearful but cease trying to escape. Flooding has many unwanted potential side effects, intentionally causes a distressed fear response, and can be dangerous to the animal and people nearby. For these reasons, ***flooding is not recommended***, and this technique is not used in this book.

Desensitization

Desensitization is a process where a stimulus is presented repeatedly in a controlled and gradual fashion.[6] Because of the gradual exposures, the individual learns that the stimulus is not meaningful, and therefore stops responding to it. Systematic desensitization requires that the stimulus be controlled in its intensity, and always kept a level where the learner does not show a response to the stimulus (Figure 3.8).

Controlling the intensity of the stimulus requires constructing a plan for graduated exposures, often called an exposure hierarchy or an exposure ladder. An exposure ladder may even contain subsets of exposures if the stimulus or end behavior is complex. Intensity of the stimulus can mean many different things. It may mean the duration the stimulus is presented, the environment in which the stimulus is presented, how loud a sound is, how soft or firm a touch is, which body part is touched based on nerve ending concentration and individual sensitivity, the distance between the learner and the stimulus, and how many factors are involved, such as equipment, odors, and more. In every case, there must be a zero-response starting point for desensitization to be effective. As an example, we can consider a possible exposure ladder and its subsets for nail trimming.

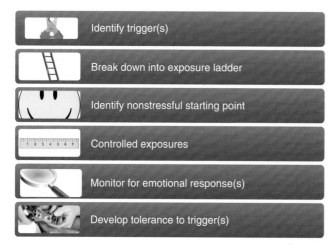

Identify trigger(s)

Break down into exposure ladder

Identify nonstressful starting point

Controlled exposures

Monitor for emotional response(s)

Develop tolerance to trigger(s)

Figure 3.8 The steps of desensitization. Desensitization is generally used in combination with classical conditioning or classical counterconditioning.

The components of the exposure ladder may look something like this:

- Touching of the target area of a toenail:
  - Touch shoulder, glide touch to elbow, carpus, paw, toe, and toenail.
- Introducing toenail clippers:
  - Touch shoulder, glide to elbow, carpus, paw, toe, and toenail while holding clippers.
- Trimming a nail:
  - While holding clippers, touch is tolerated up to and including toenail.
  - Trimmers approach nail, then approach and tap nail.
  - Trimmers approach nail, tap nail, encircle nail, and then trim a single nail.
- Trimming all nails:
  - Trimming a single nail is well-tolerated.
  - Trim two nails, then three, then four, then one entire paw.
  - Trim one paw, then begin a new paw.
  - Gradually work up to being able to trim all nails on all paws.

Desensitization takes time and patience, and the speed at which desensitization may proceed is dictated entirely by the learner. Some learners may be able to tolerate very rapid desensitization, while others require a slower approach. Desensitization will only be successful if the learner is carefully observed for signs of stress or response, and the stimulus intensity is carefully controlled. Sudden exposure to a high level of the stimulus can lead to a significant setback, or even sensitization. For these reasons, desensitization is best accompanied by counterconditioning.

Sensitization

Sensitization is a learning process in which repeated administrations of a stimulus results in the progressive amplification of a response.[6] The animal develops a stronger and stronger response over time to the stimulus (Figure 3.9). Sensitization is a risk during habituation or desensitization: instead of a lessening response over time, the response can worsen or intensify. It is crucial to monitor animals during treatment for escalations in the fear response, or visible signs of stress during treatment.

One example is sensitization to storms resulting in storm phobia. At first, a dog may only "notice" a violent storm and show a mild response. Then the dog may show a stronger response like shaking, panting, and pacing during heavy storms, and "notice" small storms. Next, the dog may have full panic during large storms, and shake, pace, and pant during small storms. Eventually the dog becomes sensitized and may have a full panic even with a small storm. Sensitization can also result in generalization of similar

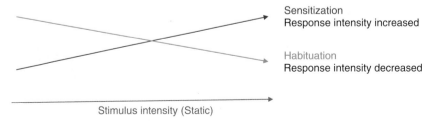

Sensitization
Response intensity increased

Habituation
Response intensity decreased

Stimulus intensity (Static)

Figure 3.9 Sensitization and habituation. When a stimulus remains the same, the learner's response may change over time.

stimuli. For instance, the storm-phobic dog may start to worry about other noises such as fireworks, the smoke alarm, a door slamming, and so on. Another example would be animals who respond progressively more strongly to having their nails trimmed with each event. At first, the dog may be mildly reluctant or withdraw his paw. Next, he might avoid all touching of the legs or feet. Eventually he may even show defensive aggression when we attempt to touch the feet. This is an example of sensitization because there is a stronger and stronger response to the same stimulus as it is presented over time.

Classical Counterconditioning

Remember classical conditioning from earlier in this chapter? **Counterconditioning** is the technique of changing an existing classically conditioned response (emotion, reflex, or secretion), and replacing it with a new response to the same stimulus.[6] By pairing a previously feared stimulus with something we know causes the *desired* emotional response, we can change the fear response to a happier one. Common tools used during classical counterconditioning include high-value treats, toys, pleasurable forms of touching, and happy verbal praise (Figure 3.10). **Classical counterconditioning** is a cornerstone of treatment for fearful animals in the veterinary setting and is almost always paired with some form of desensitization. Together, they are called desensitization and classical counterconditioning, or DS/CCC.

Classical counterconditioning is the *replacement* of an emotional response; there is no requirement that the animal performs a specific or desired behavior.[6] The goal is simply to form a pleasurable association with something he previously feared. In the examination room, every touch can predict something wonderful like a favorite treat. When the touch predicts the treat for enough repetitions, the animal should begin to anticipate something pleasurable associated with touching. If the animal is nervous about touching, the touch should be broken down into smaller segments (desensitization), and progress should be made at the animal's comfortable pace. DS/CCC to veterinary procedures will be described in depth using numerous examples.

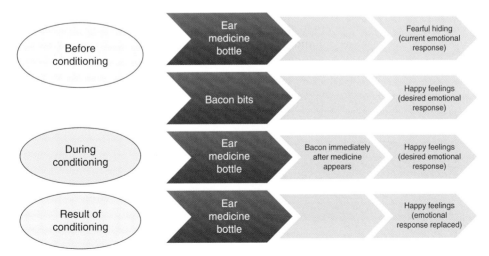

Figure 3.10 Classical counterconditioning. Counterconditioning replaces an unwanted existing emotional response with a new, desired emotional response by linking the trigger with something that prompts the desired emotional response repeatedly.

Operant Counterconditioning

Operant counterconditioning (OCC) is teaching the animal to perform a desired behavior in the presence of a previously important stimulus.[6] Some trainers call this differential reinforcement of an alternative (DRA) or incompatible behavior (DRI), while others call it operant counterconditioning or response substitution. By teaching the desired behavior, we can make it simple for an animal to comply with treatments. Furthermore, the desired behavior will not be possible while the undesired behavior is performed (Figure 3.11). For example, a dog who usually jerks his paw back when we try to touch a

(a)

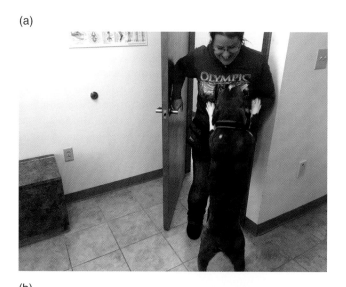

(b)

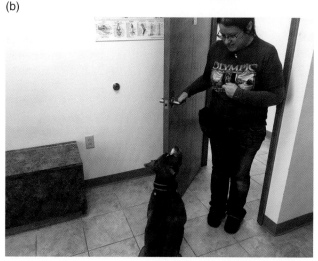

Figure 3.11 (a–b) Differential reinforcement of an incompatible behavior. This dog can't both jump up and sit at the same time. Reinforcing the sit rather than the jump will teach him to sit instead of jumping during greetings.

nail can be taught to stand and offer a paw. Standing and offering a paw is incompatible with jerking the paw away. If a cat runs away at medication time, teaching her to come to a medication station is a desired behavior we can reinforce, which is incompatible with running away (see Video 3.6). Using a training plan, it is possible to teach animals the desired behavior to cooperate for treatments.

OCC Video

In Video 3.7, an excited puppy, Lucy, barks and pulls on the leash when she sees other puppies in class. The training plan here involves classical counterconditing followed by OCC. First, we click and treat every time she looks at another puppy. This forms a classically counterconditioned response to expect something wonderful when she sees another puppy. Next, we introduce the reinforcement for looking at the handler after looking at the other puppy. This is the beginning of response substitution. The last step is to add a sit: look at the other puppy, look at the handler, then sit earns a click and treat. By dividing the skill into smaller steps, creating a pleasant response to looking at another puppy, teaching an alternate behavior, and then reinforcing an incompatible behavior of sitting rather than pulling toward the other puppies, we can teach the puppy to be more manageable and attentive. Simply asking this puppy to sit in this environment would be likely to fail; she needed additional conditioning and information to be able to understand what was expected. With a few well-timed clicks and a good training plan, this result was easily achieved.

3.4   The ABCs of Behavior

Functional Assessment

Learning terminology and theory can feel overwhelming at times. Behavior modification and training have plenty of jargon as well as scientific terminology. To help make understanding and remembering terms to physically change behavior in dogs and cats much easier, use a simple system to assess the learner's behaviors. The **three-term contingency** is used in **functional assessment**. The smallest meaningful unit of behavior analysis, the three-term contingency is not only a very useful tool but also easy to learn and remember: as easy as ABC. A is for *antecedent*, B for *behavior*, and C for *consequence*. We will look at each of these independently using a case study, "The Case of the Snapping Aussie" (see Video 3.8).

Antecedents

Antecedents are predictors of behavior. They can be distant antecedents or immediate antecedents.[5,6] Some are complex, while others are quite simple. Environmental changes or circumstances can act as antecedents, such as a drop in barometric pressure being followed by the onset of a bout of storm phobia. Other antecedents are social interactions between animals, interactions with a person, intentional antecedents like cues, tactile information, olfactory cues, and certain sounds provided by a trainer or caregiver. An antecedent is anything that precedes the behavior and predicts it will occur.

An example from Alicea:

> When I don't have to work the next day, I know I am going to stay up too late. The distant antecedent is the fact that I am off the next day; the immediate antecedent would be a *Star Trek* marathon on TV. Both are predictors of my behavior, but one is more immediate to the behavior.

Behavior

Behavior is anything the animal does: the organism's response following the antecedent.[5–7] Keep in mind that behavior cannot be changed by anyone but the organism or learner itself. We can set up antecedents and deliver consequences to make a behavior more or less likely to occur, but we cannot forcibly create the behavior. The learner is entirely in control of behavior, because behavior is simply the action of the learner. Prompts, cues, environmental setups, and more can all work in our favor in improving the likelihood of a desired behavior strengthening over time.

To modify behaviors, we must be able to observe and measure them. This means the animal is actually doing a behavior. It is not possible to observe or train the lack of a behavior. If an animal has a problem behavior the trainer wishes to decrease over time, it is important to decide what the desired alternate behavior is, and arrange the antecedents and consequences to support the desired observable, measurable behavior. Attempting to train and measure only the cessation of behavior is difficult and does not teach the desired behavior.

Consequences

Consequences follow behaviors.[5,6] Each of the quadrants in operant conditioning is a type of consequence. These consequences drive future decision making by the learner. Consequences can be environmental, intrinsic, and **extrinsic**. The consequence may be under the trainer's control, or something in the environment outside the trainer's control. Remember: the animal or learner is the one whose perception of the consequence is important.

If a dog performs a given behavior such as seeing the scale and then following treats onto the scale, then receives a favorite treat, it is likely the dog will choose to move onto the scale in the future. If a dog sees the scale, is pulled by the leash onto the scale, and then slips or scrambles while being weighed, it is likely the dog will choose not to move onto the scale in the future (Figure 3.12).

In the first example, the salient antecedents are the presence of the scale and treats. The behavior is moving onto the scale. The consequence is receiving a delicious treat. In the second example, the antecedent is the presence of the scale and pressure on the leash. The behavior is moving onto the scale. The consequence is slipping and scrambling. The same antecedent of the presence of the scale, and the behavior of moving onto the scale, resulted in two different consequences, which will drive two different behavioral choices in the future.

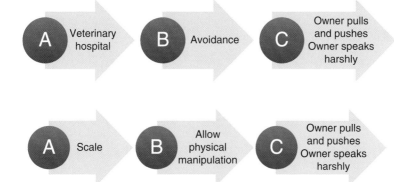

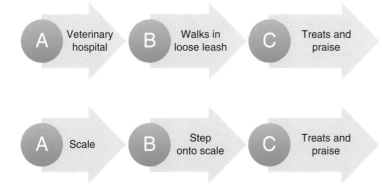

Baseline before training: Veterinary environment predicts avoidance, which are followed by unpleasant interactions.

Result after training: Veterinary environment predicts movement through lobby and placing paws on scale, which are followed by pleasant interactions.

Figure 3.12 ABCs. The antecedent, behavior, and consequence breakdown for entering the clinic and moving to the scale before and after training.

Putting It Together

When working with patients, you will find that each of the learning methods shares space. You may be using desensitization, classical conditioning, and operant conditioning in the form of positive reinforcement all simultaneously. There is plenty of overlap between these methods, which often works to your advantage as the trainer.

Video 3.8: Coco Is Fearful at the Veterinary Office

Coco is a seven-month-old spayed female Australian shepherd. When visiting the veterinary office, Coco was beginning to show more signs of fear and defensive aggression. She was very uncomfortable, (ears back, lip lick, dilated pupils, growling, and inhibited bite). Because she was restrained, it was impossible to assess her proximity preference.

When she became very uncomfortable, she would snap at the veterinary team. She was not trying to be dominant or uncooperative, but simply trying to communicate that she was fearful and defending herself against a perceived threat. To set up a training plan for Coco, we needed to understand the ABCs of her existing behavior, and the ABCs of the desired replacement behavior.

The distant antecedent to Coco's fearful defensive displays is the veterinary environment and team. The immediate antecedent is touching or attempted touching by a team member for restraint. The behavior is a distance-increasing signal: a snap, or fully inhibited bite. The consequence is the handlers stop touching Coco, and distance is increased. Because the aversive stimulus of someone attempting to hold her stops when Coco snaps, she is learning through negative reinforcement. The human correctly removes her hands (negative), and the snapping behavior is maintained or increased over time (reinforcement). Safety of the team and the patient always takes priority. Removing hands protects the team member from a bite, and Coco from flooding.

In order to teach Coco a new, desired response to handling in the veterinary clinic, we used desensitization and operant as well as classical counterconditioning. Each small step toward touch predicted a wonderful treat, which also acts to reinforce the behavior of remaining calm, and induce the desired emotional state of decreased fear. When Coco's training was completed, the same antecedent of touching by a veterinary team member preceded the behavior of allowing touch. The consequence of wonderful treats helped to increase and maintain the behavior of tolerating handling.

Example: Cat into the Carrier

When a cat is fearful of the carrier, this is often a classically conditioned response at first. The antecedent is the presence of the carrier. The behavior is entering the carrier. The consequence is being locked in the carrier, a car ride, a vet exam, some needle pokes, and another car ride. This consequence will likely result in a decrease in the behavior of entering the carrier, and an increase in the behavior of running away even at the sight of the carrier.

The current behavior of running away from the carrier and the emotional response of stress and fear can both be changed. The desired replacement behavior would be for the cat to enter the carrier on her own. The desired emotional response is pleasure when the cat sees the carrier. To break down the training picture, the antecedent would be the presence of the carrier. This antecedent is probably best accepted if the carrier is a normal part of everyday furniture, stored in one of the cat's living areas, near the cat's play area or climbing tree, or the like.

Using desensitization and classical counterconditioning, the emotional response to the carrier can be improved over time. At first, the carrier may need to be covered or far away, then closer and closer, until the cat is happy near the carrier and willing to interact with it. Once the emotional response is improved, the behavior of following treats or a toy into the carrier, or even walking into the carrier as a trick, can be trained. The antecedent of the owner presenting the carrier would be followed by the behavior of the cat walking into the carrier. The consequence would then be receiving treats or a toy after entering the carrier, likely increasing the behavior of entering the carrier and decreasing the behavior of running away.

3.5   Fundamental Training Skills

When it's time to start training patients that need help, you'll need a training plan. It is imperative that we focus on positive reinforcement. While implementing your positive reinforcement training, keep in mind that capturing, shaping, desensitization, classical conditioning, counterconditioning, and response substitution will all be occurring at the same time. Focus on developing the desired behavior, and monitoring and assessing the patient's responses, emotions, and progression of learning.

Training Plans

Alicea shares an example:

> My two biggest fears are the dentist and flying. I finally found a dentist who understood how to help me. She takes the time to educate me completely and get me ready before visits. She sends out videos of what the procedure will look like from beginning to end before my appointments, and checks with me throughout the appointment to see how I am feeling. I found the videos helped me greatly. I also took an online course for people afraid to fly. They too used video to explain everything from start to finish. What both approaches did was take the mystery out of what was happening. They explained every sound and sensation and what to expect in a linear fashion. Where am I going with this? Your training plans should be like the educational video. It prepares your patient before he is expected to do the behavior perfectly or at least willingly. Each step in your shaping and desensitization will paint the picture of the ultimate goal.

Predictability and understanding are a good way to build trust and decrease fear, anxiety, and stress. By using a training plan, taking a systematic approach, observing the animal's responses during training, and going at a comfortable pace for the animal, we can provide veterinary care that is much less upsetting to our patients and often use little or no physical restraint. Before a trainer is ready to make a training plan, both the trainer and the animal need to have a good grasp of the fundamentals of training.

Rewards and Reinforcement

Rewards matter. When starting a session with an animal, it's important to choose a reward that actually *reinforces* behavior. While you won't know if the reward you choose is truly reinforcing until you see the pattern of increased behavior emerge over time, you can often predict based on common preferences what an animal might find reinforcing for a given behavior. Developing a reinforcement hierarchy will be important when training new behavior with an animal. For instance, Alicea's Jack Russell terrier, Piper, loves to tug. She will learn a new behavior or respond to cues for the opportunity to tug on a toy. In a very distracting environment or when she is nervous, tugging has little value and food creates a better response. Monique's Border collie, Rye, prefers tugging in exciting environments, a tennis ball for moving behaviors, and food for calm behaviors. Invest some time to learn what the animal wants, then develop an order of preference. Learning the effects of, and preferences for, different types of foods, treats,

Table 3.1 Example reinforcement hierarchies: Individual preference and the context of the situation will determine how patients are motivated.

Animal	Situation	High value	Medium value	Low value
Border collie (no prior fear of grooming)	Nail trim	Steak	Kibble	Tennis ball
Border collie	Recall away from squirrels	Tennis ball	Tug toy	Steak
Terrier	Going for a walk around squirrels	Cheese	Kibble	Tug toy
Terrier	Learning a new trick at home	Tug toy	Cheese	Kibble
Kitten	Learning a recall inside the house	Feather toy	Cream cheese	Cat treats
Kitten	Physical exam at the veterinary hospital	Cream cheese	Canned cat food	Feather toy
Cat	Learning to go into a carrier at home	Cream cheese	Kibble	Feather toy
Cat	Learning a medication station	Cream cheese	Facial stroking	Cat treats

toys, touching, and other forms of potential reinforcement will speed up the training process, and give the trainer plenty of tools in the toolbox when challenges emerge. Table 3.1 shows examples of reinforcement hierarchies.

Questions about Rewards

What if a pet likes treats, but won't eat them?

We should ask a few questions: is the animal hungry, or already satiated? Is the animal relaxed enough to accept food? Is the food a desirable treat for this animal? How can I make the environment calmer and less stressful to improve food acceptance? Is the behavior I am trying to train too difficult? It's important to persist in trying to help animals feel comfortable enough to take treats, experimenting with a variety of different types of treats, reducing environmental stress as much as possible, and exploring other reinforcement strategies until you determine what works best for each individual pet. Figure 3.13 is a quick reference for improving food acceptance.

Training Tip: Counting Calories

Make sure your patient is receiving the right number of calories per day. Overfed or overweight pets will be undermotivated and won't work as hard for food rewards.

If you can use toys, petting, and praise, then why use food?

Not all rewards are equally reinforcing for certain behaviors. There are two types of reinforcers we will concentrate on for this guide: primary or unconditioned reinforcers, and secondary or conditioned reinforcers. Primary reinforcers are naturally reinforcing

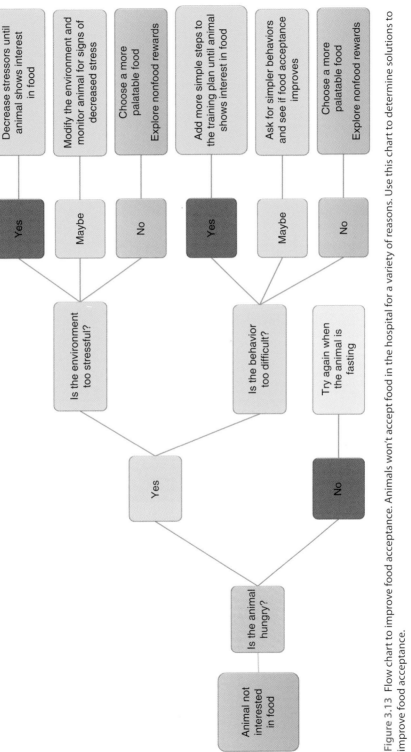

Figure 3.13 Flow chart to improve food acceptance. Animals won't accept food in the hospital for a variety of reasons. Use this chart to determine solutions to improve food acceptance.

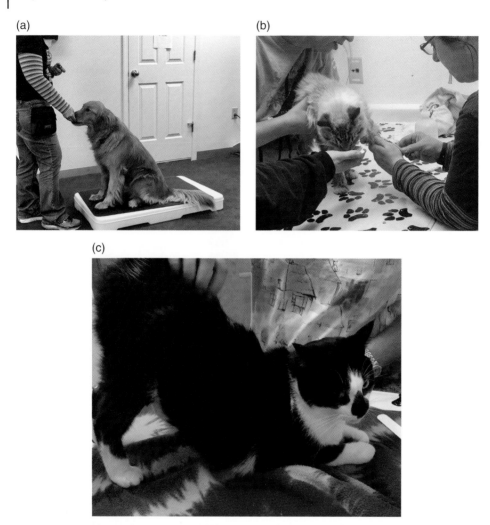

Figure 3.14 (a–c) Primary reinforcers include food for most dogs and cats. Many cats also like this type of tactile interaction, and will work for tactile reinforcement.

for the animal and do not require any training. Some examples of primary reinforcers include: food, water, reproductive opportunities, and shelter. Animals will naturally expend effort and work to access primary reinforcers (Figure 3.14). However, even primary reinforcers are not equally valuable to an animal. For example, hiking an extra five miles to have a bigger salad might not be so appealing, but doing so for some delicious ice cream may be more motivating for some people. Remember that what is reinforcing is up to the learner and not the trainer. The value of an item can also change as availability and access to the item change. For instance, if I am a millionaire, I will probably not be motivated to do an hour of work for $20. I can have money anytime I'd like it.

Novelty and "other peoples' cookies" can play a role. Clients should always come prepared with a favorite treat such as chicken, steak, canned food, or cream cheese from home. These are familiar items to the animal. In the hospital, we might offer something that seems lower value like cat treats, and the animal may prefer it simply because it is novel. The key to success is to be flexible and ready to change based on what the animal prefers during any given session.

Note: When we use the word reinforcer, *what we mean is something intended to provide reinforcement for a given behavior. If the behavior gets stronger over time, we will know reinforcement is successfully occurring.*

What about secondary reinforcers?
Secondary reinforcers derive their value from being paired with primary reinforcers in a predictive relationship. For this reason, secondary reinforcers are also referred to as conditioned reinforcers.[6,7] For example, the clicker is a secondary reinforcer. A click is heard; a delicious treat appears. The click predicts the treat often enough that the click becomes a conditioned reinforcer because it consistently predicts the appearance of a primary reinforcer. You will know the click has become a conditioned reinforcer when the animal responds to the click by anticipating a treat (orienting to the handler, raised ears, eager facial expression, tail wag, etc.).[6]

Money is a good example of a conditioned reinforcer for most people. We can't eat money; it won't quench our thirst or give us shelter. However, money can predict the presence of a primary reinforcer because it can be exchanged for food, water, shelter, and much more. Think about how you feel when given a bigger paycheck or handed money for your birthday. Money is reinforcing because it leads to receiving the primary reinforcement of your choice, which triggers happy feelings. Money is only valuable if it retains its purchasing power, and in reality, the value of money is somewhat arbitrary and can change. If the money you received for your paycheck became like every other piece of paper and you could no longer use it to buy anything, it would hold little value for you. This concept is important because it applies to the trainer's task of maintaining the value of secondary reinforcers. A click is a way for an animal to "purchase" a treat. It's important for the click to continue to allow the animal to buy treats; otherwise, the click will lose its value and the animal will be less motivated to try to earn clicks.

Other types of conditioned reinforcers used by trainers are praise from a familiar and preferred person, toys, and known cues. A cue such as "sit" can become a conditioned reinforcer when trained using positive reinforcement. The trainer gives the cue "sit," the pet sits, and a treat is given. The cue "sit" begins to predict a behavior that is linked to a primary reinforcer. Through classical conditioning, the cue "sit" and the behavior of sitting can cause a positive emotional change in the animal similar to what they experience when receiving the treat that generally follows. After the cue is well understood by the learner, it can reinforce and mark the previous behavior like a clicker would.[7,8] Using behaviors as conditioned reinforcers is how we chain multiple behaviors together and give only one food treat at the end. Table 3.2 shows a comparison between some primary and secondary reinforcers for most animals.

Building Behaviors: A Good Foundation

A complex behavior like reading requires us to first learn the foundations of the alphabet, how to make words, what the words represent and mean, and how they connect together forming sentences and paragraphs. As we become more advanced readers, we learn that similar words or chains of words can have different meanings depending

Table 3.2 Primary and secondary reinforcers: Primary reinforcers require no learning history, while secondary reinforcers have been classically conditioned to be reinforcing because they predict primary reinforcement.

Primary reinforcers	Secondary or conditioned reinforcers
Food	Money (humans!)
(and food acquisition sequences)	Click
Water	Verbal bridge
Reproductive opportunity	Known cue
Shelter	Location, odor, or object
Rewarding without *any learning history*	*History of* predicting *primary reinforcers*

upon context. Just like learning to read, to become a proficient veterinary trainer you'll need a good foundation made up of many component skills. Good trainers understand learning theory, and also correctly observe and accurately interpret communication from their animal learners. Constructing training plans, using marker-based training, using lure-reward training, and applying basic behavior modification techniques are all critical materials for building a well-rounded veterinary trainer.

Like the trainer, the animal needs a good foundation as well. For an animal to engage in veterinary training, useful foundation behaviors include paying attention or attending to the trainer, responding to the clicker or other marker, responding to cues, stationing, and targeting. A good foundation for trainer and learner will help your team build complex behaviors. If you want to teach complex behaviors, you will need to train the foundation behaviors separately first.

Foundations for the Trainer

Methods

For veterinary training, we suggest three main methods of applying positive reinforcement to teach an animal a behavior: lure-reward training, shaping, and capturing. Luring is suitable for basic or simple behaviors and behaviors that are needed only once, while shaping is more appropriate for complex behaviors and serial behaviors. Shaping and capturing have been detailed earlier in this chapter, and we will discuss luring here.

Lure-reward training uses strategic movement of food lures to encourage an animal into a certain position or location.[6] A few examples of luring include encouraging a cat to follow a treat out of a carrier, or a dog to follow a treat while walking to the exam room. The position of the lure, what is being used to lure the animal, and the eventual training goals for the behavior all combine to determine the proper luring technique. Because the lure can easily become part of the cue for the behavior, it is important to limit the use of luring to select appropriate situations.[6]

Correct luring will show the animal where to go or what position to assume, be physically comfortable for both the trainer and the animal, deliver a primary reinforcer once the animal is in position, and allow for the addition of a cue during the training process (Figure 3.15). Luring the animal means delivering treats at a rapid enough rate that the animal makes progress in the correct direction, while staying interested in the process. A good lure is like a pact or a promise. When the animal gets to the point where the lure

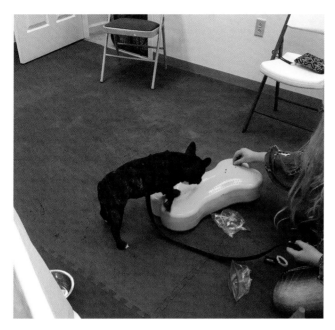

Figure 3.15 Correct luring means the animal is willing to move freely toward the treats, and they are positioned so the animal will perform the desired behavior.

was offered, a small amount of food is given. One analogy is that luring is like following stepping stones across a stream. Each stepping stone is a stopping point along the path where reinforcement happens while you're on your way to the goal of getting across. If the animal is reluctant to make forward progress, assess the animal and the environment. Assuming the animal's overall stress level is low and the environment is sufficiently welcoming to allow training, animals who won't follow the lure are communicating they are confused or lack motivation. In these cases, we can refer back to the stepping stone analogy. Either the stepping stones are too far apart, they are trying to span a gap that is too wide (we are asking too much of the learner), or the reward found when the learner gets to the stepping stone is not sufficiently desirable (Figure 3.16).

Video 3.9 shows two methods of luring a puppy onto the scale. In the first example, the puppy is reluctant to move. The environment is not overly stressful, and the puppy is motivated by the tasty canned food, but the "stepping stones" are too far apart. Each time the puppy gets to the point where the lure was presented, the treat is pulled further away before he can eat anything. The puppy is reluctant to move because the rate of reinforcement is too low, and the distance he must move for a small bite of food is constantly changing. In the second example, the video shows the correct way to lure the puppy. The trainer makes the lure increments closer together, and assures the puppy is allowed to eat something at each stopping point.

Modeling
With **modeling**, the trainer uses a body prompt or light touch to demonstrate what we want the animal to do.[8] Modeling a paw lift or hug is a quick way to get started training a behavior, but the training plan needs to include a plan to fade the prompt over time.

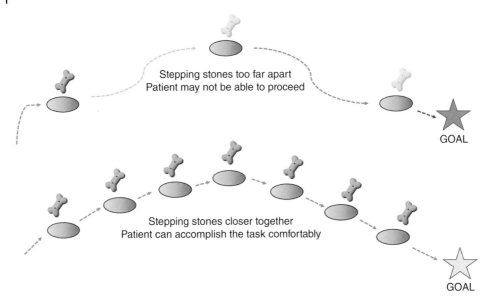

Figure 3.16 Stepping stones. When luring, shaping, or trying to achieve any goal behavior, the process must include enough incremental steps so the patient can achieve success. Assure each step feels comfortable and possible for the learner. Keep the stepping stones close enough together for the patient to successfully reach the goal behavior.

Because modeling is one of the few times we will start by touching the animal, it is important that we closely observe the animal's response to touching and assure there is no unwanted sensitization.

Whether using lure-reward or modeling, the best practice is to use the smallest amount of prompting necessary to elicit the behavior. Gradually, use smaller and smaller amounts of prompting until the animal is offering the behavior without the prompt. As with other methods, modeling uses a combination of positive reinforcement with desensitization and classical conditioning or counterconditioning to achieve the result of a happy patient performing the desired behavior at the end of the training process.

 Modeling can also be used to teach acceptance of touch, like in Video 3.10. Millie has already leaned her consent behavior of stationing (see Chapter 7). Notice when she is on the station, Alicea uses modeling to teach a physical exam. She first names the behavior and then reaches for the body part, showing Minnie the behavior by touching her. Minnie doesn't lift her own ear or leg but gives consent by remaining on the station and not moving away. She is reinforced with food for every body part that is touched, and she is learning through cues what to expect.

Cues and Cueing

If we remember the ABCs of behavior – antecedent, behavior, and consequence – we know that behaviors follow antecedents, and consequences follow behaviors. A cue is also called an antecedent or **discriminatory stimulus**.[3,6,7] A cue is something that comes before the behavior; it is a clue to the animal that "if you perform this behavior, reinforcement may occur." Essentially, a cue is a signal to the animal that reinforcement is available for a certain behavior. Cues can be intentional or accidental, and can be environmental or handler-based. Cues that come from the trainer are generally signals, words, or a combination of both. Animals are usually more sensitive to signals and body movements or postures, while people communicate primarily with words. In the training videos, you will note the technicians speak frequently, but this is largely for the benefit of observers. A majority of the cues we give in these videos are body language and gestures or signals.

For an animal to understand a cue, it needs to be consistent. The same signal, gesture, word, or combination should mean reinforcement is available for one consistent behavior. As the trainer, we need to be mindful of what we would like the cue for a behavior to be, and make sure we present the cue in the same fashion for every repetition so it is easy for the animal to understand what we mean. There are a few behaviors that require the animal to tolerate variety. For example, auscultation requires the stethoscope in several different areas, and not every veterinarian may perform auscultation in exactly the same way. The "cue" for auscultation in this case may be the presence of a stethoscope and a word rather than a precise body movement or signal.

Sometimes it is impractical to teach the final cue from the beginning of the training process. For example, say we want a dog to step onto the scale with the verbal cue "mat." In the early stages, the cue for this may look like me standing near the scale and pointing, which is a prompt most dogs would understand. To change the cue, we can use a process called a *cue transfer*. The cue transfer is simply giving the new cue, then giving the current cue, waiting for the behavior, and then reinforcing the behavior (Figure 3.17). For this example, we would say "mat," then we would stand in the prompt position and point. After a few repetitions, the animal will offer the behavior preemptively in response to the new cue, rather than waiting for the initial cue. Once this occurs, the new cue can be used exclusively.

Video 3.11 shows an example of fading prompts and cue transfers using the example of targeting. Here, a target is used as the cue for Kyrie the cattle dog to move to the target and lie down. Once she understood how to move to the target, it was placed on the table to introduce the concept of getting onto the table. Once she was reliably getting onto the table for the target, the trainer performed a cue transfer so that her hand became the cue to get onto the table, rather than the target.

Video 3.12 shows another example of a cue transfer, teaching a dog to go to her mat when someone knocks at the door.

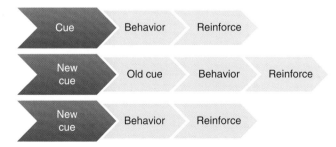

Figure 3.17 Cue transfer steps. A known behavior can be placed on a new cue by using the new cue to predict the old cue. After several repetitions (more repetitions for more complex behaviors), the learner should begin to offer the behavior in response to the new cue.

Table 3.3 The four factors of stimulus control.

The four factors of stimulus control	
• When the cue is given, the behavior occurs promptly.	• When the cue is absent, the behavior does not occur.
• When the cue is given, only the cued behavior occurs and no other.	• When a different cue is given, the behavior does not occur.

Lastly, cues are related to stimulus control. Establishing stimulus control is an advanced training skill, and may be useful in some circumstances or unnecessary in others. **Stimulus control** means the behavior occurs on cue, only on cue, not in response to a different cue, and not when the cue is not being given (Table 3.3).[7,8] Often animals will offer behaviors that the trainer has reinforced in the past, even when the behavior has not been cued. Some behaviors are desirable when the trainer or owner wants the behavior, but problematic if the animal offers them at the wrong time or in the wrong context. One example is if a trainer teaches a dog to "speak." Barking may be desirable when the cue is given, but if the dog offers barking off-cue to try to obtain reinforcement, or "push the cookie button," it can present problems in the wrong context. When you see stimulus control mentioned in this book, it is for practical reasons rather than academic training reasons. *Refer to the Appendix for details on achieving stimulus control.*

Foundations for the Learner

Like the trainer, the learner will need a few foundation behaviors to achieve the best results for veterinary training. These foundation behaviors are helpful for almost every veterinary patient, and we suggest teaching them as a part of the first few visits with any new patient, young or old. These foundation behaviors can easily be used to prompt new behaviors and improve communication between the veterinary team and the patient in a variety of different situations. The foundation behaviors are nose targeting, paw targeting, stationing, response to cues, and attention to the handler.

Nose Target
Nose target refers to the behavior of teaching an animal to touch her nose to something. Sometimes the target is the trainer's hand, or a target stick, or a specified object like a training disc or paper marker (Figure 3.18). Nose targeting is useful because it allows the trainer to change where the animal is, direct the animal to orient a specific way, and show the animal how to move from point A to point B without using a food lure and without touching the patient.

Teaching Nose Targeting: Canine   First, assess the environment. Work in an area that is not too distracting, and where the learner feels comfortable. Remember: if stress levels are too high, it will be difficult for the dog to focus and learn something new. Assure the

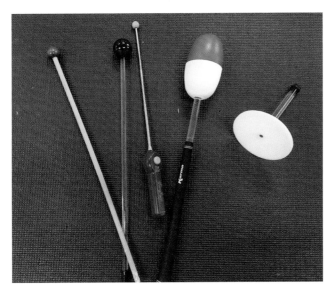

Figure 3.18 A variety of objects used to train nose targeting.

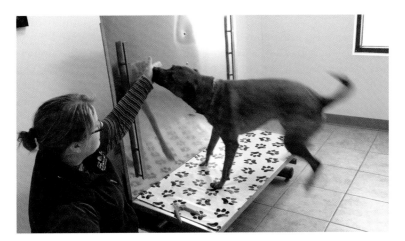

Figure 3.19 This dog is targeting the trainer's hand with his nose.

dog is motivated and likes the rewards you have, but keep your hands empty and away from your pockets. Hold a clicker in one hand; the opposite hand should be empty. Most dogs are naturally curious and have a terrific sense of smell. Open your empty hand and show your palm to the dog, reaching gently toward her. The curious dog will generally sniff or lick your hand (Figure 3.19). Click the instant you feel contact with your hand to capture the nose target, and then reach into your treat bag for a reward. The click should occur while the dog is in contact with your hand, and the treat will follow afterward. Repeat this process for several repetitions, until the dog participates without hesitation.

Once the dog is happily targeting one hand, change hands and reinforce her for targeting the opposite hand as well. Next, assure the dog is touching the hand quickly when it is presented. Offer the hand target, and count in your head to five seconds. If, within five seconds, the dog has not touched, remove access to your hand target for five seconds, and then try again. The goal is for the dog to promptly touch either hand. Once the dog is promptly touching either hand, you may wish to introduce a verbal cue for this behavior in addition to the visual cue of the flat palm. Many trainers use the word "target" or "touch" for this behavior. At the same time the palm is presented, speak the verbal cue as well so the dog has a chance to learn both cues for this behavior.

Training Tip: Getting the Target

Some pets may be distracted, or have trouble noticing the hand target at first. Wait until the pet is looking at you, then present your hand. The movement of your hand will often entice the animal to investigate, leading to a nose touch.

Once the dog is willing to touch either hand, and do so promptly, begin offering the hand target in a variety of different positions: high, low, left, right, forward, and backward. Reinforce the dog with a click/treat for every touch, while teaching the dog to reorient to find the hand target that has been offered.

Video 3.13 shows Alicea demonstrating the introduction to nose targeting with a puppy in the examination room. The puppy is simultaneously being introduced to the idea of targeting as well as charging the clicker. After only a few attempts, the puppy is very focused on the trainer's target hand, and he is showing a visible response when he hears the click, telling us he is starting to understand the click is meaningful and predicts something pleasant. This puppy also shows how dogs are focused on movement. By rapidly moving her hand to a new location, the trainer generates interest in the hand and encourages the puppy to explore the idea of moving to reach the hand target.

Teaching Nose Targeting: Feline   As with dogs, assure the environment has few distractions, and is a comfortable place for the cat to work. It is important to be sure the cat is hungry and interested in the treats you're offering. Like dogs, cats are curious, but they tend to explore by sniffing and cheek rubbing rather than licking like a dog would. Offer an empty hand toward the cat, with one finger outstretched. Click for any interest shown in your finger, and then treat after the click. If the cat does not immediately make contact with your finger, make this a shaping exercise. At first, any interest in your finger earns a click and treat. The next steps are moving toward your finger and making contact with your finger. Once the cat will target one finger, as with dogs, change hands and offer a finger on the opposite hand.

After the cat is touching a finger on either hand, you may wish to introduce a verbal cue. In addition, begin offering the target finger in different locations such as up, down, left, right, forward, and back. Some cats may prefer to target an object rather than the trainer's hand. A target stick is useful to teach nose targeting for these individuals (Figure 3.20).

Video 3.14 shows Alicea teaching a kitten nose targeting. In this kitten's first training session, he is touching a target stick and accepting food readily. The kitten quickly advances from just touching the target stick to moving toward the stick to touch it.

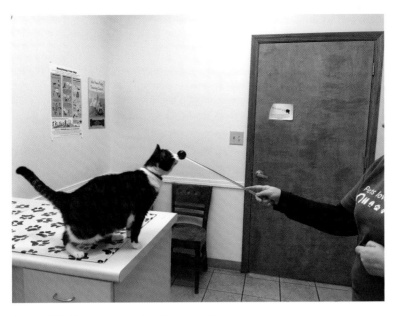

Figure 3.20 This cat is targeting the stick with her nose.

During the second session, Alicea generalizes nose targeting to a new location by teaching a finger target. In this case, after a few repetitions, the kitten is readily offering the targeting behavior in exchange for a click and some play.

Alternative Targets   Hands and fingers are just the beginning as far as nose targeting goes. Target sticks, large spoons, tongue depressors, and pens are all examples of alternative targeting items. In some cases, it is not appropriate to allow the patient to approach the trainer's hands. In other cases, the patient may be small, and reaching out to offer your hand will cause the trainer to loom over the patient in a counterproductive way. In addition, target sticks can be easier to use when having a patient follow, as this keeps the hands free for a leash, a clicker, and treats. Target sticks can also be used through kennel run doors or cage bars for cases in which protected contact is desired between the animal and the trainer. This technique is used in zoos and aquaria around the world every day.

Video 3.15 shows using a target stick to teach a cat how to move into a carrier. The target stick is a good choice for this behavior because it can reach into the carrier without blocking the opening like a hand and arm would.

Following a Target   For both dogs and cats, once the pet understands how to touch a target in a variety of orientations, the pet is ready to learn to follow. Following a target can be used to move onto the scale, from the floor to a mat or the exam table, from the exam room to the treatment room, and anywhere else you need the patient to move.

It is important for the animal to be able to easily meet criteria when introducing this exercise. Remember the stepping stone analogy for luring. The same principles apply to following a target. Only ask the animal to move a few inches or a few steps at first, and proceed at the rate the animal is prepared to move.

First, present the target, whether it is your hand, a target stick, a spoon, and so on. As the animal shows interest in the target, move it an inch or two so the animal moves forward to reach the target. When the animal moves toward the target and approaches it, click and treat. With subsequent repetitions, gradually move the target greater distances for the animal to follow prior to reinforcement.

Video 3.16 shows using target following to encourage a terrier in and out of a cage in the hospital. This dog already understands targeting and following, so this is a good example of how useful these foundation behaviors can be.

Training Tip: Targeting, Not Treating!

Remember, targeting means the animal is *choosing* to touch a target with a specific body part. Never place food on the target. Placing food on the target teaches the animal to eat food, not to make the choice to move to the target and touch it.

Paw Targeting

Paw targeting is the behavior of placing a paw on a designated target, such as the trainer's hand, a target disc, a mat, a washcloth, a towel, a paper target such as a sticky note, and so on. Paw targeting using a small mobile target is useful in getting animals to move around in the exam room, onto the scale or examination table, and into and out of kennels or carriers, and even to present paws for nail care training and peripheral venous access training.

Teaching a Paw Target   Work in an area that has few distractions, and assure the patient is interested in the rewards you have to offer. Select something to use as your paw target, such as a FitPAWS® target disc, a small section of a yoga mat or rug, or a small fabric or paper target such as a sticky note (Figure 3.21).

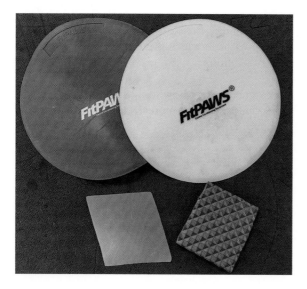

Figure 3.21 A variety of objects used to train paw targeting.

When working in a small area, capturing is often effective at teaching a paw target. Place the target in the area where the dog or cat is likely to be moving around. When the pet accidentally steps on the target, click during the instant the paw is touching the target, then follow the click with a treat. After a few repetitions, the animal will begin intentionally touching the target with a paw. At this point, you may wish to add verbal cues and/or signals as cues in addition to the presence of the target, to allow flexibility later in your ability to determine when the animal will perform this behavior.

Shaping can also be used to teach paw targeting through successive approximations. When shaping, the target will be presented and the animal will earn clicks and treats for progressively approaching the desired behavior. For example, at first simply looking at the target would earn a click, then moving one step toward it, then moving several steps toward it, then raising a paw near it, and finally touching the target with part of a paw and the entire paw. At this point, you may wish to add a word and signal to use as the cue for paw targeting.

In both cases, once the animal is offering the paw target behavior promptly when the target is presented or the cue is given, begin moving the target small distances, so the animal learns to traverse the distance to complete the target behavior. As with the process of teaching following a nose target, keep the distances short at first, and make sure the animal can easily achieve the goal. Gradually, the animal can be asked to move greater distances, and even up onto a platform or table, and in or out of a kennel or room.

Whether the capturing or shaping method is used, realize that many patients have a dominant paw preference, much like most people have a dominant hand for writing. If there is a particular paw you would like the animal to use for this behavior, select it early and only reinforce for the selected paw. In advanced training situations, it may be helpful to have an animal offer more than one specific paw. Patients are capable of learning to differentiate between each paw as a distinct targeting behavior with training.

Training Tip: Paw Targeting
Paw targeting is a foundation behavior for many more complex skills, including nail board training. Nail board training is an alternative to nail trimming. Refer to Chapter 7 for more information.

Video 3.17 demonstrates training a terrier to touch a FitPAWS target with her paw. Once she learns the desired behavior is touching the target with a paw, Alicea can begin moving the target around to show the dog how to follow the target and placer her paw in Alicea's hand. Video 3.18 demonstrates paw target training with a feline patient.

Paw targeting is an example of a skill that may benefit from stimulus control, or at least partial stimulus control. Some owners may object if their pet is offering the paw target behavior in new places or new situations, such as pawing at the owner to seek attention or request food. As a technician, it might be difficult for me to clean an animal's ears if he is trying to give me his paw in my hand. Most animals will learn the proper context for this behavior, but if the animal is offering the behavior at inappropriate times, an effort to achieve stimulus control may be helpful. (See "Stimulus Control" in the Appendix.)

Body Targeting

Body targeting refers to teaching the animal how to move to a target and stand, sit, or lie down on the target. Body targeting is very useful because we can have the animal move around the room, onto the exam table, onto the scale, to a medication or treatment station in the clinic or at home, in and out of the kennel, to their bed to relax out of the way at home, and much more. While body targeting can be trained using lure-reward training, we are advocates of using capturing and shaping to train this behavior for best understanding on the part of the patient, and for the most durable behavior under mild stress such as during veterinary procedures.

Teaching a Body Target: Canine　Work in an area with few distractions, and assure the animal is interested in your rewards in that environment. Choose a target that is large enough the animal can simultaneously place at least two, and preferably four, paws on the target. Introduce the mat, bed, rug, or other target, and wait. At first, click for any interest in the target such as looking at it, sniffing it, moving toward it, or moving around it. Gradually increase the criteria to leaning over the mat, stepping onto the mat with part of a paw, then a whole paw, then more than one paw, and eventually all four paws. Once the dog is moving to the target reliably, ask for a known behavior with a strong history of reinforcement such as a sit or a down on the mat.

Placement of reward is important when teaching body targeting. Some animals do best when receiving the treat on the mat, while others benefit from the treat being tossed away from the mat to reset for another attempt. Pay attention to the learner: is he reluctantly placing a paw on the edge of the mat? Give the treat at the mat. Is he running to the mat and lying down, and it is difficult to get him to move away for more practice? Give a small treat at the mat and another tossed away from the mat to reset for the next repetition.

When shaping, we need to find the balance between rate of reinforcement, increasing and decreasing criteria, and getting understanding from the animal without confusion. Finding the balance can seem overwhelming at first! Take the time to experiment and practice. You won't do any harm by practicing, and you'll build your skills and your confidence.

The rate of reinforcement needs to remain high enough that the animal can sustain interest during the session, but low enough that the animal is willing to offer "improvements" on the behavior. If looking at the target earns 20 clicks and treats in a row, the dog will be unlikely to try to move toward the target. Why would he, when simply looking is enough? However, if the criterion is too difficult, such as expecting the animal to place four paws on the mat immediately, the rate of reinforcement will be too low and the dog may lose interest, or try offering other known behaviors instead of exploring this new skill.

Video 3.19 shows Alicea introducing body targeting to her newly adopted Greyhound. The goal behavior is for this dog to go to the mat and lie down. Alicea begins by clicking and treating for interest in the mat, such as sniffing it or looking at it. Next, she clicks and treats when the dog moves toward the mat. Once he has moved toward the mat, he places a paw on the mat, earning a click and treat. Next, the criterion is increased to placing both front paws on the mat for a click and treat, then all four paws. When the dog is reliably offering all four paws on the mat, Alicea clicks for going to the mat and then gives a cue for "down." In this example, the cue for down should reinforce the behavior of going to the target, and the treat should reinforce the behavior of lying down on the target. (This is only true when there is a good, strong

reinforcement history for the behavior of "down.") After a few repetitions, the dog will begin to anticipate the down when he gets to the mat, and the down cue is no longer needed. Alicea has now built a new behavior, body targeting the mat in the down position, and she will introduce a new cue that means "target the mat with your body in the down position."

Stationing

The station is the area where most veterinary training and reinforcement will occur. Cues and reinforcement happen at the training station. For veterinary training, we are focusing on specific behaviors that are useful for veterinary care and animal husbandry. In most cases, we do not need to generalize these behaviors to a variety of locations or contexts, so making use of stationing is helpful and productive without compromising training goals. Choose a station that makes sense for the animal and the trainer, as well as the owner if the behavior such as taking medication will need to be repeated at home. In the clinic, common choices for a station include a rug, mat, yoga mat, nonslip exam table cover, low platform, or exam table (Figure 3.22).

Stationing allows the animal to consent for a procedure and choose to engage in training, or send a clear signal to the trainer the animal is uncomfortable and not ready for what is being asked. By giving the animal some control in this situation, we can reduce stress and anxiety, decrease fear, increase comfort, and increase the animal's ability to cooperate.

Video 3.20 shows the difference between learner control and trainer control. Look for the changes in body language with two dogs who have both been training to accept nail trims using desensitization and classical counterconditioning. Both dogs do hold still and accept nail clipping. However, when offered the nail board (Figure 3.23) to file their own nails, they become more relaxed and loose in their movements. These dogs are more calm and comfortable when they are in control of the procedure (nail board) rather than when the trainer is in control of the procedure (nail clip).

It is easy to accidentally begin moving toward an animal out of impatience to complete the task. Keep the station pure and safe, and respect that it is consent or lack of consent. Coming to station is a way for the animal to tell you she is ready to participate. Staying on or at station is the animal's way of saying she is comfortable with what is occurring. If the pet is reluctant to stay on station, assess yourself, the animal, as well as the environment; consider if what you are asking the animal to do is too difficult based on her learning history and current situation.

To introduce the station, work in an area with few distractions, and make sure the animal is interested in your rewards in this environment. Choose a station that is easy to define visually (tactile cues work for blind patients), and make sure you have a good definition in your mind. In general, we suggest the definition of four paws on the station, and the patient shows interest in the handler. The patient should be free and unrestrained. If the patient is wearing a leash, it should be dragging, but we highly recommend the leash be removed. (If the patient requires a leash for safety reasons, the patient is not yet ready to learn stationing.) To encourage the animal to station, use another foundation behavior such as nose targeting to a hand, paw targeting to a mat, or body targeting to a mat that is at the station. You may also use shaping, as was described for body targeting, but if the animal has a good target behavior, targeting will be faster than shaping to teach the station.

(a)

(c)

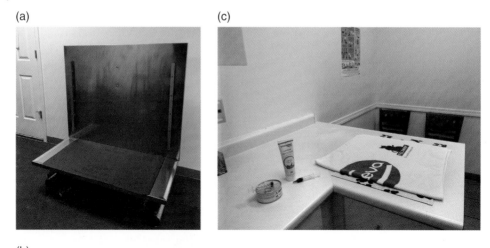

(b)

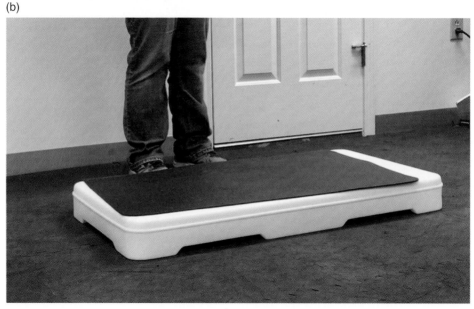

Figure 3.22 (a–c) Three different stations. These are just a few examples among many possibilities.

Once the animal is at the station, having followed a target or been shaped to choose to go there, interaction and training begin. Coming to the station signifies an opportunity for considerable reinforcement. Reinforce every 1–2 seconds at first simply for remaining at the station. If the animal chooses to leave the station, don't respond and make sure you stop giving treats. When the animal shows interest in the trainer again, use a target behavior to invite the animal to return to the station. If the animal is reluctant to return to the station, assess the animal, yourself, and the environment for sources of increased fear or stress.

When the patient is comfortable remaining at the station for several seconds in a row, begin introducing nonthreatening touching while the animal is stationed. For dogs, this

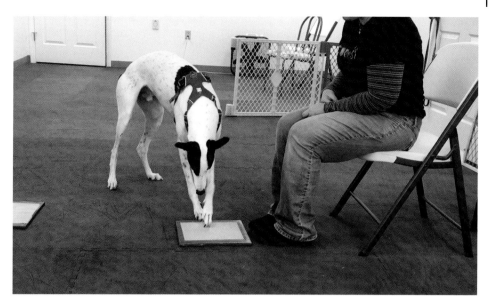

Figure 3.23 Nail boards are an alternative to conventional nail trimming.

generally means a low rub on the chest between the front legs, or a gentle stroke along the sides. For cats, this generally means a light touch along the cheek, or a gentle stroke along the back. Help the animal learn the "touching game." Touch, click, treat. Touch, click, treat. Each touch predicts a click and a treat. Very rapidly, the animal will begin happily anticipating touching. This method uses a combination of operant conditioning, desensitization, and classical conditioning to encourage a positive emotional response as well as the behavior of remaining at the station for touching. Remember: if the animal chooses to move away, that is her way of showing she is overwhelmed or uncomfortable, and a signal to the trainer to reassess the plan before trying again.

Video 3.21 shows a kitten's first exposure to the idea of stationing. In this example, a combination of luring, capturing, and shaping is used to encourage the kitten to station. As Alicea consistently rewards him when he comes to the blanket, he begins to return to the blanket more frequently.

Stationing is an incredibly useful foundation behavior for both dogs and cats, as long as the trainer remembers to respect the animal's right to move away if he is uncomfortable. Forcing a pet onto the station, restraining him at the station, or preventing him from leaving when he wants to will diminish the pet's ability to trust the veterinary team. Less trust means less success. Refer to Chapter 7 for more stationing examples.

Adding Duration

Nose targeting, paw targeting, body targeting, and stationing are all wonderful foundation behaviors. However, there are few medical tests and treatments we can accomplish in 1–2 seconds. Over time, it will be necessary to teach an animal how to hold the target position or station for gradually longer periods of time, until the release or end-of-behavior cue is given. Because a click is a signal that the behavior has been completed, adding duration is often as simple as *briefly* delaying the click. Using the example of a body target, ask the animal to move onto the target and down, then mentally count "One banana." Click and treat at the end of the held position, and then gradually begin adding time before each click.

Tasks that always increase in difficulty can be demotivating for some learners. When adding duration, gradually ask for longer behaviors, but intermittently sneak shorter durations in as well. For example, if we are training for a 10-second hold, we may reinforce after 2 seconds, 5 seconds, 1 second, 10 seconds, 3 seconds, 9 seconds, 15 seconds, 11 seconds, 4 seconds, and 7 seconds. This is an average of 7 seconds of holding over 10 reinforcement events, which is close to the goal of 10 seconds without wearing out the learner by continuously asking for more and more difficult repetitions.

Attention to the Handler

Working with an animal on foundation behaviors will naturally cause her to check in with the handler more often. By teaching the animal that attending the handler is also a way to earn clicks and treats, we are giving the animal a reliable way to earn rewards between exercises, and establishing a way to begin training again if for some reason the patient opts out or becomes distracted. To teach attention to the handler, simply be aware of the patient's attention and focus. Anytime the patient checks in with the veterinary team member by looking at or turning toward them, click and treat. The animal should begin checking in more and more frequently with the veterinary trainer as the reinforcement history for this behavior grows. (This is also a great life skill for pet owners and their pets out in the world!)

For example, if a dog has come to the station and we are practicing ear handling, and the dog leaves the station, this is an opportunity to reinforce attending the trainer. As soon as the dog turns toward or looks at the trainer, click and treat. Now the dog will have returned his attention to the trainer and is showing he is likely ready to return to work. Invite the animal to station again and see what happens: usually an animal who is attending the trainer is ready to try again.

Video 3.22 shows rewarding a young dog for attending the handler and following her. Notice the trainer moves around, which gives the puppy an opportunity to repeatedly orient toward the handler, showing she is ready to work. The trainer waits for the puppy to reorient and pay attention after each treat, then reinforces for attention.

Refer to the "Puppy Class Syllabus" in the Appendix for more detailed information about attention training.

Conclusion

Every interaction we have with a patient is a training opportunity. Unlike punishment-based methods, positive reinforcement and marker-based training carry no real risk when training mistakes happen, and will not result in harm to the patient if errors occur. The concepts introduced in this chapter of classical conditioning, desensitization, classical and operant counterconditioning, and operant conditioning will all combine to make more advanced training plans for patients in subsequent chapters. By understanding the science of learning and applying the science, we can provide patient-centered veterinary care. Mastering these skills empowers technicians to provide the very best-quality care available for patients and clients.

References

1 Friedman, S. (2010) What's wrong with this picture? Effectiveness is not enough. *Association of Pet Dog Trainers Journal.* March–April, 41–45.

2 Kalat, J. (2010) *Introduction to Psychology.* Independence, MO: Cengage Learning.

3 Skinner, B.F. (1945) The operational analysis of psychological terms. *Psychological Review.* 52 (4), 270–278. https://doi.org/10.1037

4 Herron, M., Shofer, F., and Reisner, I. (2009) Survey of the use and outcome of confrontational and non-confrontational training methods in client-owned dogs showing undesired behaviors. *Applied Animal Behaviour Science.* 117 (1–2), 47–54.

5 Skinner, B.F. (1966) *The Behavior of Organisms.* New York: Appleton-Century-Crofts. (First published in 1938)

6 Shaw, K., and Martin, D. (2015) *Canine and Feline Behavior for Veterinary Technicians and Nurses.* Ames, IA: John Wiley & Sons.

7 Ramirez, K. (1999) *Animal Training: Successful Animal Management through Positive Reinforcement.* Chicago: Shedd Aquarium Society.

8 Pryor, K. (1999) *Don't Shoot the Dog: The New Art of Teaching and Training.* New York: Bantam.

4

Successful Visits: Environment and Protocols to Prevent Fear and Stress

Prevention is always the best medicine! Why treat what we can prevent? In general practice, we spend a great deal of time preventing common diseases and parasites, and setting up preventive nutrition protocols, educational protocols, and testing protocols for monitoring health. Preventive medicine can and should also encompass behavioral health, inside and outside the veterinary hospital. Compliance is a sizeable issue in veterinary medicine, and clients who own fearful pets are less likely to present them for wellness or interventional care, because of perceived stress.[1] Setting up the environment and basic protocols to prevent fear and stress in the veterinary hospital will prevent problem behaviors for many patients.

Pets of all ages can benefit from prevention, not just puppies and kittens. Preventive behavioral care geared toward making veterinary medical treatment easier and safer for people and pets as well as toward keeping pets in their homes and protecting against relinquishment starts with making a plan. Remember, fearful behaviors tend to intensify with time and repetition, especially when no intervention is provided. This chapter is dedicated to preventing exam room worries before they start. Every interaction, from our first meeting with a client and patient, is an opportunity for success. While some animals may need extra training and medical management even when we've done everything we can for prevention, many patients will respond well to these preventive protocols. For those animals who need intervention, Chapters 5 through 7 will outline interventional plans suitable for every patient.

4.1 Setting Up for Success: Before the Visit

At Home

Imagine every time you get into the car, you go to the dentist's office or to pay your taxes. You might learn to have an unpleasant opinion of car rides because they predict something unpleasant. It's easy for dogs and cats to learn to fear travel in the car, harnesses, and carriers if they always predict something unpleasant. Puppy and kitten owners as well as new clients should be advised to make wearing a harness and collar fun. Clients should take time to teach pets to enjoy short rides in the car by visiting enjoyable locations such as drive throughs with dog treats, or a favorite park. Cat carriers should be kept in the main living area of the cat's quarters, incorporated with a normal resting place such as a cat tree, and paired with enjoyable items like catnip, cat treats, and special toys. Treating cat carriers with a pheromone product such as Feliway® prior to travel often helps cats relax.

Help clients know what kind of cat carrier is best. A hard-sided carrier with quick-release clips on the sides and back is easiest to use at the veterinary hospital. These carriers are safe and secure, and quick and easy to disassemble for veterinary visits. Soft-sided carriers can be useful as well, especially for cats who already have a conditioned emotional response to a hard-sided carrier, or cats who require sedation for examination. Figure 4.1 shows a cat carrier that has clips which are easy to open for veterinary visits, and provides safety during travel.

If a dog is so fearful of car rides that the owner has difficulty loading him, or a cat is so concerned about a carrier she disappears as soon as she sees it, intervention rather than prevention is needed. Desensitization and classical counterconditioning will help, and sometimes in-home coaching is needed to help clients learn to load pets into the carrier or the car. Prior to veterinary visits, some pets need a supplement or prescription to help them relax and ease loading. In severe cases, consultation with a **veterinary behaviorist** may be indicated.

Making the Appointment

Our first opportunity to set up a successful appointment is when the client calls. A knowledgeable receptionist is crucial for successful patient visits, particularly for first-time clients and patients. Clients should be instructed to make sure their pets (both dogs and cats!) are hungry when they come to the clinic, and to bring some of the pet's favorite treats and a toy if the pet loves toys. Ideally, one pet should visit per appointment to reduce any social pressure in the exam room. One exception to the single-pet guideline would be bonded dogs who are allies and are more anxious when they are separated but more relaxed when they visit together. Anxiety can be contagious between pets, and one nervous animal can spread the nervousness through the whole

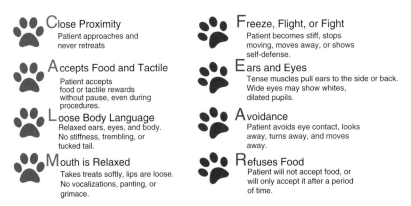

CALM or FEAR?

Close Proximity
Patient approaches and never retreats

Accepts Food and Tactile
Patient accepts food or tactile rewards without pause, even during procedures.

Loose Body Language
Relaxed ears, eyes, and body. No stiffness, trembling, or tucked tail.

Mouth is Relaxed
Takes treats softly, lips are loose. No vocalizations, panting, or grimace.

Freeze, Flight, or Fight
Patient becomes stiff, stops moving, moves away, or shows self-defense.

Ears and Eyes
Tense muscles pull ears to the side or back. Wide eyes may show whites, dilated pupils.

Avoidance
Patient avoids eye contact, looks away, turns away, and moves away.

Refuses Food
Patient will not accept food, or will only accept it after a period of time.

Figure 4.1 CALM or FEAR? Patient assessment is complex and fluid. Use these basics as a good starting point.

Table 4.1 Checklist for scheduling appointments.

Appointment scheduling checklist
☐ Check medical record for notes.
☐ Schedule special needs patients accordingly.
☐ Remind client to give any necessary medications.
☐ Remind client to fast pet.
☐ Remind client to bring favorite treats and toy.
☐ If necessary, plan for client to call from parking area.
☐ Ask for any questions or concerns before the visit.

exam room. Also, multiple pet visits prolong the time each pet must spend in the hospital. Lastly, each veterinary team member can only devote his or her full attention to one pet at a time, including monitoring for and reducing fear and anxiety. If multiple pets must be scheduled, make a plan to keep the pets as comfortable as possible. Cats should each have their own carriers rather than being transported together. Dogs need to be leashed, and may even be seen one at a time rather than simultaneously if a safe nonstressful arrangement can be made for each dog to wait while the other is being treated.

If a dog needs extra space and is stressed by the presence of other dogs, there will be a note in the medical record indicating this need. The receptionist should schedule this dog's appointment at a quiet time when no other dogs will cross paths with the dog who needs space. Sometimes arranging for these clients to call from the car on arrival rather than coming into the lobby, or arranging a separate entry through a side door, will help reduce stress before the visit as well. Table 4.1 provides a checklist for scheduling appointments.

4.2 During the Visit

Patient Assessment Tools

Assessing the patient is a key in determining what interactions will be most appropriate. This chapter is all about prevention, and Chapters 5 through 7 will each be dedicated to progressively more fearful, anxious, or stressed patients. To determine the patient's stress level, we suggest the following evaluation criteria:

Dogs:
1) Food acceptance
2) Body language
3) Proximity preference.

Cats:
1) Food acceptance and/or toy acceptance, tactile
2) Body language
3) Proximity preference and exploration versus hiding.

During each interaction, every team member should be familiar with these three criteria, and monitor them throughout the visit. As discussed in Chapter 2, changes in food acceptance, body language, and proximity preference are cues to the veterinary team about the animal's emotional state and comfort level. The goal of prevention is to set up an environment and set of protocols such that the animal's stress level remains low or absent as a baseline in the hospital whenever possible (Figure 4.1 provides a quick reference graphic for patient assessment).

Dr. Colleen Koch has developed a useful algorithm for making decisions about what treatments are appropriate at each stage of a visit, and taking into consideration wants versus needs (Figure 4.2). This algorithm provides helpful suggestions in a succinct manner. The concepts introduced in this algorithm will be revisited repeatedly. The vast majority of what we do in regular practice are wants. Needs are lifesaving measures for unstable patients. Temperature measurement, vaccination, conscious x-rays, oral examination, and lab work on healthy or chronically ill patients are all examples of wants. Wants can always be rescheduled, postponed, or abbreviated for patient well-being. A training plan and possibly medical intervention can be set up, and then the patient can be better prepared for treatments in the category of wants.

The Lobby: Setup and Equipment

Make sure there are plenty of tasty treats available in the reception area, in addition to any treats the owner may have brought along from home. In a perfect world, patients spend very little time in the reception lobby, but in case of waiting the lobby should be set up and marked with separate areas for dogs and cats. Figure 4.3 shows an example of a reception desk with a selection of treats above the scale, and a reception area divided into smaller waiting areas. These areas can be separated quite simply by using the positioning of chairs into two distinct seating areas, planters, displays, solid benches, half-walls, screens, and more. An elevated area to place cat carriers is helpful, rather than placing carriers on the floor or the owner's lap. Pheromone diffusers can be used, and if music is played it should be relaxing.

Social contact should be minimized in the waiting area. Social stressors such as inter-acting with other pets or with strangers can increase anxiety and decrease the patient's ability to cooperate for treatments. Dogs should be on a short leash (no retractable leashes) attached to a harness, martingale, or flat collar. Cats should be in a cat carrier or harness and leash. Prong collars, choke collars, and electronic collars are not appropriate for the veterinary environment. The client services team should monitor pets and people, to assure no inappropriate interactions occur, and interrupt inappropriate inter-actions if they begin by escorting the client to a different area or to an exam room. Table 4.2 shows a checklist to begin setting up the lobby.

The Entrance: Dogs

Our first interaction with the patient begins in the parking lot or the reception area. A properly trained team member should greet the patient and client. It is crucial for the client services and reception team to be trained in the evaluation tools of food acceptance, body language, and proximity preferences. It can be easy to accidentally overwhelm mildly nervous dogs with good intentions. The receptionist may choose to offer treats and a greeting if the dog is comfortable and happy to receive them, and should discontinue any interaction that increases the dog's stress level. The receptionist should direct the owner to an examination room, or to appropriate waiting area until an examination room is ready.

Algorithm for handling patients

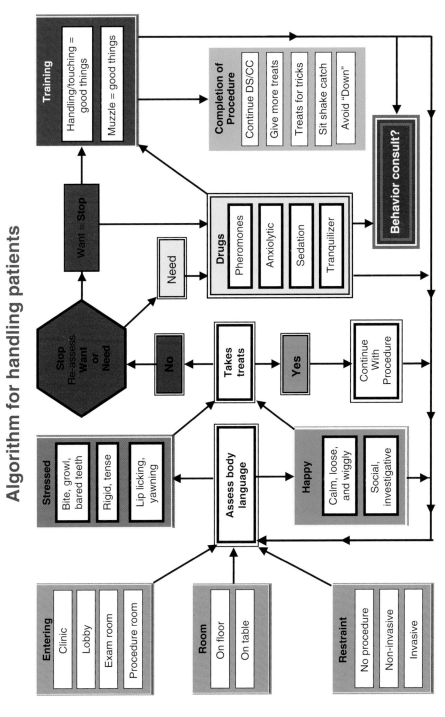

Figure 4.2 Patient-handling plans. This detailed algorithm outlines planning patient care based on patient assessment, medical therapies indicated, and tools available. *Source:* Courtesy of Colleen Koch, DVM.

(a)

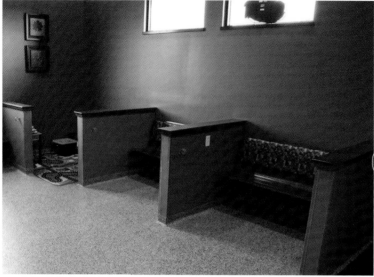

(b)

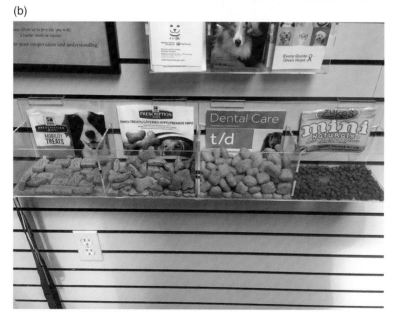

Figure 4.3 Reception area. (a) Divided waiting area at Mile High Animal Hospital. (b) Wide variety of treats in the reception area at Mercer Island Veterinary Clinic.

The Scale

Have you ever wondered why dogs hate the scale? Unlike us, it has nothing to do with the number on the display. Consider the scale from a dog's perspective. A stranger or your owner pulls you to a wall or a corner, and pushes you onto a slippery, unstable surface. Every time this unpleasant experience happens, it is followed by the even more

Table 4.2 Preparing the lobby or reception area.

Reception and lobby checklist

- ☐ Nonslip surfaces
- ☐ Variety of treats
- ☐ Pheromone product diffusers
- ☐ Calming music (if any)
- ☐ Separate areas by species, or visual dividers
- ☐ Elevated area for cat carriers
- ☐ Loaner leashes and carriers available
- ☐ Signs reminding about appropriate collars

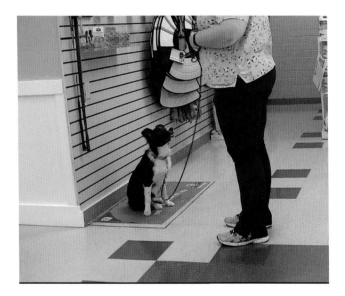

Figure 4.4 Keep a variety of treats near the scale, and assure the scale has a nonslip surface.

unpleasant experience of going into the exam room for temperature measurement, needle pokes, and a probing and prodding examination. If we consider it from the dog's point of view, it makes sense. When going onto the scale is an unpleasant experience that predicts an even more unpleasant one, classical conditioning will cause the dog to become frightened of the scale itself.

To correctly weigh a dog, we must abandon the pushing, pulling, and the owner scolding, "Sit. SIT. SIT!" We need to assure the scale is as inviting and comfortable as possible for the dog. The scale should have a nonslip surface and should be in an open area when possible. Many clinics, including the clinics of both authors, have recessed scales so the top is flush with the floor, making the transition easier for dogs. Keep treats near the scale, and use a treat trail to encourage dogs to walk onto the scale. If the dog already has the foundation skill of following a target, hand targeting, or body targeting on a mat, these skills can also be used to make weighing a breeze (Figure 4.4). If the dog is mildly anxious, having the owner make the treat trail is sometimes helpful.

Carefully observe and coach the owner when necessary, as sometimes owners will escalate out of frustration or embarrassment when a dog is difficult to weigh, worsening the experience for the dog.

Video: Weighing a Large Dog

In Video 4.1, you will see a new technician working to get a large dog onto the scale. The greyhound is friendly, but confused about what he is supposed to do and reluctant to step onto the scale. Eventually, the technician lifts the dog by herself onto the scale, which presents a risk for injury as well. During the second attempt, the technician uses a treat trail to encourage this dog to move onto the scale. Notice how she positions her body to make the path onto the scale obvious without looming over the dog, and allows him to move at his own pace. The dog freely follows the treat trail on a loose leash, and has a positive experience on the scale. This takes less than half the time of physically manipulating him onto the scale, and causes none of the associated stress. After a few examples like this one, most pet owners can walk their own dogs onto the scale in a gentle and effective manner.

The Entrance: Cats

In contrast to dogs, who usually will wish to greet the reception team, most cats will be in a carrier, and many cats experience a higher level of stress at the veterinary hospital. The client services team should greet the client in a calm and friendly manner, and either invite the owner and cat directly into an exam room, or provide a quiet area in the lobby to wait until a room is ready. Many owners will try to lift the cat carrier by the handle, which allows the carrier to swing in an unsettling way. When inviting cat owners to the exam room, the client services representative may wish to carry the cat herself, or instruct the owner to carry the kennel from the bottom using both hands to avoid swinging movements that will make the cat feel unsteady.

The Exam Room

Moving into the examination room can be frightening for some animals, especially those who have had negative experiences in the past. To make the exam room as inviting as possible, follow these simple tips. First, when possible, have species-specific exam rooms. Particularly cats will benefit from having their own room. Interspecies social signaling is decreased, which can reduce stress levels for some patients. If a cat is very stressed in the feline exam room, cleanse the room thoroughly after that cat's visit to minimize pheromone signals left behind. Use pheromone diffusers or other preparations in each exam room. Provide nonslip, comfortable surfaces for patients, including on the floor, on the exam table, and anywhere else the pet is expected to spend time. To avoid patients getting trapped or stuck in tight spaces, select closed-bottom furniture and position it so there are very few tight hiding places. Store a variety of delicious treats of different flavors and textures in the exam rooms, and means to administer them such as dishes, paper plates, sturdy plastic spoons, tongue depressors, syringes, and pretzel rods. Keep a few likely favorite toys in the rooms as well, such as tennis balls, squeaky toys, and a cat fishing pole. Store the basic equipment you're likely to need during visits in the exam room, or gather all the equipment needed for a patient at the beginning of the visit to minimize the need to relocate the patient or repeatedly enter the exam room.

Figure 4.5 shows examples of a variety of nonslip surfaces in the exam room, and suggestions for a variety of treats, toys, and treat delivery options to keep in each room. Table 4.3 provides a checklist to begin setting up the exam room.

(a)

(b)

(c)

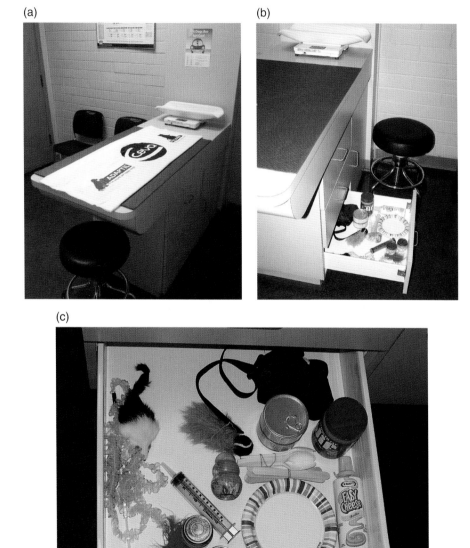

Figure 4.5 (a–c) Nonslip surfaces should be provided in the exam room, as well as a variety of treats and toys close at hand.

Table 4.3 Exam room preparation checklist.

Exam room checklist
☐ Nonslip surfaces on floor and table
☐ Wide variety of treats
☐ Toys, including food-dispensing toys
☐ Treat delivery tools (spoon, target, and pretzel rod)
☐ Pheromone products
☐ Calming music (if any)
☐ Separate areas by species, or visual dividers
☐ Syringes, needles, blood tubes, etc.
☐ Otoscope, ophthalmoscope, etc.
☐ Scissors and zip ties to open/close carriers if needed
☐ Body language posters
☐ Passive educational materials about care planning
☐ Signs reminding about appropriate collars

The Exam Room Experience: Dogs

Dogs should be encouraged to move around the room and explore. Larger patients should be allowed to stay on the floor or a low platform, while smaller patients might be more comfortable on the table. Select an area to work based on the dog's preferences. Food acceptance, body language, and proximity preferences will tell you where the dog feels most comfortable.

When collecting a history, the technician should be multitasking. When possible, remove the dog's leash and allow him the freedom to explore, approach, or retreat. Use treats tossed around the room to help dogs explore and feel comfortable, and offer food to assess food acceptance. Make note of the dog's body language and proximity preferences to you, as well as which treats the dog prefers. When the history is completed, if the dog is comfortable being approached and touched, collect the vital signs as appropriate.

With any touching, begin in a less sensitive area before moving to a more sensitive one. For example, when palpating a femoral pulse, begin touching along the shoulder, then glide your hand down the back to the flank and then to the medial femoral area. During touch, assess and reassess the dog's body language and food acceptance. Pair touching with something wonderful! In many cases, the owner can be helpful if instructed in proper techniques for giving food, where to place the food, how quickly to give the food, and to notify you if the dog stops eating. The same principles can be used to measure body temperature. Begin touch in a less sensitive area, and make sure the touch predicts wonderful treats. Minimally displace the tail, and then measure the temperature. If the dog is not comfortable with temperature measurement, save this procedure until the end of the visit, or omit it if the information is not truly necessary.

In Chapter 2, Figures 2.6 and 2.7 showed a gradient example of relative sensitivity in dogs and cats. The lightest shaded areas have the lowest concentration of nerve endings, while darker shaded areas contain a higher density of nerve endings. The darkest shaded areas will be the most sensitive to touch for most patients, while the lightest areas are the least sensitive. One exception is the cheek of the cat, which is rich with nerve endings, but a pleasurable area when touched for many cats.

Video 4.2 shows measuring the temperature of a puppy on her first visit. Not only is this the puppy's first visit, but also the clients are first-time dog owners. The owner has been instructed to keep treats near the puppy's nose, keep the treats stationary, and provide treats repeatedly until the procedure is complete. The technician begins touch along the puppy's back, then slides to the rump, and gently moves the tail prior to measuring the puppy's temperature. This puppy is learning many things in these brief seconds: how to enjoy being on the table, touching predicts wonderful things, temperature measurement is associated with wonderful things, and how to hold still for treats. The client is also learning: that the team cares about this puppy's experience, the technician loves puppies, the puppy can learn to like veterinary care, and how to properly deliver treats to encourage a dog to hold still.

Once the history and vital signs measurement have been completed, it is time to round the veterinarian. When providing the medical history, also provide information about the dog's emotional state, preferred working area, treat preference, and how he responded to touch. Good communication helps each team member save time, improves efficiency, and improves the patient experience.

Plan the physical examination like every other aspect of the visit: to build the most comfortable experience for the patient. To improve cooperation and decrease fear and anxiety in the exam room, start with the least invasive touches, such as checking the skin and coat, lymph node **palpation**, and auscultation. Gradually work up to more invasive touching, such as the abdominal palpation, ear examination, oral examination, or any painful areas. During each phase of the exam, teach the dog that touches predict wonderful treats, working to classically condition a positive emotional response to examinations. Monitor the dog continuously for changes in food acceptance, body language, and proximity preferences. If signs of stress and anxiety emerge, pause the exam and make a handling plan to improve the dog's experience during the exam and any future visits.

Video 4.3 shows a brief example of Monique working with Border collie puppy Kestrel to introduce a few components of her physical exam. Notice that each touch predicts a delicious treat.

During regular exam visits, many dogs need to give a blood sample or allow vaccination. Applying the same principles used during the exam will help dogs feel comfortable and cooperate. Vaccinations and venipuncture should be paired with wonderful treats for every patient, and the procedure should be done gradually. For example, before giving a vaccination, touch a nonsensitive area, touch the injection area, pinch the skin tent lightly, pinch more firmly, and finally inject. Each step of the process should predict a small wonderful treat. This injection process in a comfortable dog will take about 10 seconds, and will teach the dog that injections are nothing to fear. In many cases, the owner can assist with feeding treats during this process.

Video 4.4 shows a Labrador mix puppy receiving her first vaccination. Her owners have been instructed how to give small delicious treats throughout this process. She wiggles a small amount because she is following the treats, but does not even notice her vaccinations. This is a good example of a prevention protocol for vaccinations in young dogs.

Venipuncture can be slightly more complicated because the dog must hold still enough for the technician or veterinarian to access a vein, whereas subcutaneous injections like vaccines do not need to be nearly as precise. Many owners do not understand this important difference, so take time to explain precisely what the dog will need to do and what your job is before you begin. As with the vaccination process, allow the dog to become comfortable with light stabilization, then with holding off the vein, followed by alcohol application, touching and pinching the site, and then finally venipuncture. Each step in this process should predict wonderful treats, and many dogs will stand still for venipuncture if the owner or a team member distracts them with food.

In Video 4.5, we see a senior dog named Lucy being vaccinated and giving a blood sample. She is standing on a nonslip mat, and a pet owner is feeding treats at nose level. A technician gently stabilizes the dog for the vaccination. She is supporting the dog without restraining her, but has one hand ready just in case the dog responds to the needle sensation. A second technician touches the injection area and gives the vaccine. This dog responds to the needle sensation by turning to look at the injection site, but rapidly returns to eating. A few seconds later, the team works together to collect a blood sample. The same technician is stabilizing the dog and occludes the vessel, while a second technician gently touches the area, pinches to assess the dog's response, and then collects a small blood sample. The dog eats treats during the entire procedure, and does not respond at all to the needle sensation this time. Her positive experience during the vaccination made the blood sample collection go more smoothly.

The Exam Room Experience: Cats

Cats should be allowed the opportunity to explore the exam room, or be allowed to hide if they prefer to do so. Hiding is a stress-reducing coping mechanism for cats, so let the patient show you what makes him most comfortable. Once the cat has been invited into the exam room, the owner should place the carrier on the floor, bench, or exam table and open the carrier door. Treat a towel with Feliway, and place it over the carrier, leaving part of the door opening uncovered so the cat can choose to come out. Ideally, the owner will bring this towel from home. Place a small amount of highly palatable food such as canned food, cream cheese, or a butter pat outside the kennel door to encourage the cat to explore.

Many cats will choose to exit the carrier and explore after a few minutes. Be patient, and discuss the history questions with the owner while you allow the cat to acclimate. This is a good multitasking opportunity. During the history, assess the cat's food acceptance, body language, and proximity preferences. While talking with the owner, use the time to offer treats and toys for cats who will explore. If the cat chooses to remain in the carrier, this is a sign of stress. Do not force the cat to exit the carrier, but rather plan a single handling event for these cats: vital signs, exam, and weight.

For cats who choose to exit the carrier, many can be lured onto the scale with a small amount of the same palatable food offered to encourage them to come out. For those who choose to stay inside the carrier, gently disassembling the carrier around the cat and allowing him to stay inside where he is comfortable will help reduce anxiety. Refer to Chapter 2 for signs of moderate and severe stress in cats, as these indicate the need to pause and make a new plan.

Sometimes pet owners bring carriers with difficult bolts or broken clips, or held together with zip ties. Keep nail clippers and zip ties in each exam room to disassemble and quickly reassemble carriers in disrepair. Figure 4.6 shows a carrier with quick-release clips, which are the easiest type to disassemble during veterinary visits.

(a) (b)

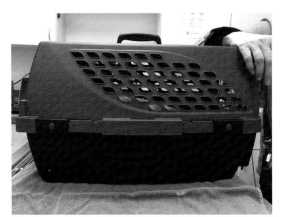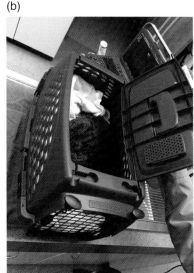

Figure 4.6 (a–b) Using carriers with quick-release clips and alternate openings simplifies visits for cats.

Video 4.6 shows a kitten during her first and second appointments in the clinic. The beginning of the video is the kitten coming out of her carrier for canned food at the start of her very first appointment. She is a little nervous but comes out to get the canned food. The second half of the video shows the same kitten three weeks later. Even though this cat received vaccines during her first visit, she came right out for food treats again at the second visit. Her first associations with the exam room are yummy food treats and gentle handling. Allowing the kitten to come out at her own pace and pairing the experience with something wonderful helped her make a positive emotional response. Working hard to help kittens feel comfortable is an investment in the future: cats who feel comfortable in the veterinary clinic.

Once the history and weight are completed, it is time for vital signs measurement for cats who come out of the carrier. Just like with dogs, begin touches in less sensitive areas before moving to more sensitive areas. For example, when palpating a femoral pulse, begin by touching along the shoulder, then glide your hand down the back to the flank, and then to the medial femoral area. Continue to monitor the cat's response to you. Is she still interested in food and facial petting? What about her body language: is it relaxed or more nervous? Is she trying to move away, or willing to stay nearby? Use these assessments and reassessments to guide your handling plan, and listen to the cat if she asks you to stop. As with dogs, pair touching with something wonderful when possible. The owner can be instructed how to help give food. Teach the owner how to keep the cat interested. Some cats will eat while you measure their temperature. Begin touching the cat in a less sensitive area, working down to the rump. Minimally displace the tail, and then measure the temperature. If the cat is uncomfortable with temperature measurement, save this procedure until the end of the visit, and ask the veterinarian to assess whether temperature measurement is crucial information during this visit.

When the history and vital signs are complete, or the history and assessment show the cat should only be handled once, it is time to round the veterinarian. When providing the medical history and presentation, team members should remember to provide information about the cat's emotional state as well. Whether the cat is accepting food and play, how the cat responds to touch, and if the cat is choosing to hide should be communicated along with health information. Good communication makes it easier for the veterinarian to create an efficient handling plan prior to interacting with the patient.

A good physical examination is brief and pleasant, and does not require restraint. Work where the cat is comfortable. This may be the floor, the owner's lap, the exam table, the bottom of a carrier, or even hiding under a towel.

Figure 4.7 shows several places a cat might like to be examined: on the table in a soft bed, in the bottom of the carrier, or on the owner's lap. Begin the exam with gentle

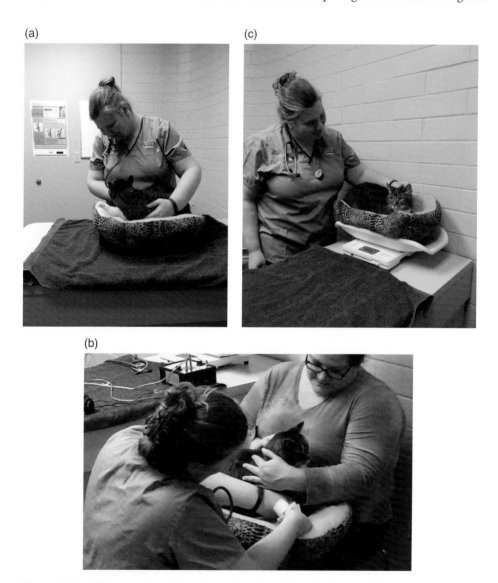

(a)

(c)

(b)

Figure 4.7 (a–c) Choose a place where the cat is comfortable, such as in a soft bed or on the owner's lap. *Source*: Courtesy of Landon.

touching in the least sensitive areas, and work to more sensitive spots. The oral examination and any painful areas, or areas noted in the record as stressful in the past, should be reserved for last. For cats who will accept food and toys, each portion of the exam should predict something pleasant happening, to encourage the cat to develop a positive emotional response. Many cats are more sensitive than dogs to the introduction of touch. Once contact is established, try to maintain at least one point of physical contact with the cat, using a gentle glide with the grain of the fur, or lightly swapping hands, to avoid startling the cat. Watch for signs of startle such as a flinch, the skin crawling, or moving away from newly established touch.

Vaccinations, venipuncture, and cystocentesis are often part of wellness visits for cats. In the chapters for Level One, Two, and Three training (Chapters 5–7), we will discuss providing these procedures for cats. Many kittens and some adult cats will allow these procedures using distraction techniques like those discussed for dogs.

The Trip Home: Cats

The visit to the veterinary hospital isn't over when the cat owner receives the receipt and goes home, especially for multicat households. Social groups of cats develop a group odor as well as a group pheromone profile. This group odor is one way that cats identify one another as members of the accepted social group. When one cat visits the veterinary hospital and then returns home, sometimes other cats at home may act aggressively toward the returning cat. To prevent this, apply Feliway to the cat carrier before the client leaves the clinic, and advise the client to use something with the home scent to rub on the cat when she arrives home. Place the newly arrived cat in another room like a bedroom for a few hours while they acclimate to being home again, and gradually reintroduce the cats under supervision. Intercat aggression secondary to reintroduction can have lasting emotional effects for both cats, so prevention is important. A single fight can lead to long-term problems with intercat aggression.[2]

4.3   Happy Visits and Other Preventative Planning

Happy Visits

Happy visits are a great way to prevent fear of the veterinary hospital. Happy visits are free of charge for the client, and have a great value for the patient, client, and veterinary team. Any patient is welcome to come for happy visits to form or maintain positive emotional responses about the veterinary clinic. In a happy visit, the patient should visit the hospital, and have a pleasant interaction with a team member such as receiving treats and a quick play session. Depending upon the layout of the hospital and current caseload, having the dog hop on the scale or walk into an exam room for a few treats are also great experiences during happy visits.

The purpose of happy visits is to show the puppy or dog (rarely, cats) they can visit the veterinarian, have a great experience, and then go home. These visits help tip the scales in favor of good experiences at the hospital rather than worrisome ones. Animals with a history of negative experiences at the vet, including recent surgery or treatment for injuries, and those who display moderate stress signals will often benefit from happy visits. Hillview Veterinary Clinic even instituted a Happy Visit Punch Card. When the client comes for five happy visits, they receive $5 off their next veterinary care appointment. Positive reinforcement works on clients as well as patients! However, if an animal is showing moderate or severe stress before approaching the clinic or in the lobby, happy visits may not be a good starting point, and repeated exposures without more planning could do more harm than good. Dogs with moderate or severe stress should be signed up for medical intervention and training visits rather than passive happy visits.

Happy visits help add value to your practice in the eyes of the client as well as the patient. Public perception is that the veterinary office is a frightening place, and that animals fearing the veterinary clinic is normal. Happy visits are one way to show clients that pets can learn to like the veterinary hospital, and how important pet well-being is to the veterinary team. When clients see the veterinary team's deep and genuine love and compassion for patients, it will help bond clients to the practice. For animals showing moderate or severe stress during attempted happy visits, this is an opportunity to open a dialog about scheduling training appointments prior to the next veterinary care appointment. Figure 4.8 shows a puppy interacting with a team member during a happy visit.

Puppy and Kitten Visits

Puppies and kittens present a wonderful opportunity for the veterinary team: the opportunity to make a great first impression. The great opportunity to make a good first impression is also a big responsibility. Puppies and kittens are in a critical developmental stage during their juvenile wellness visits. The developmental stages include **fear periods**, where young animals easily become fearful of novel things. It makes sense, if

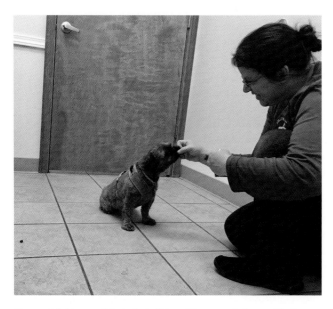

Figure 4.8 Happy visits help build positive associations with the veterinary hospital.

we consider the wild counterparts of our canine and feline pets. Novel things can be dangerous, and learning to be cautious of them is a functional fear response, as we discussed in earlier chapters. If puppies and kittens learn the veterinary clinic is a place where frightening things happen during this developmental period, fear of the veterinary clinic can last a lifetime. To help puppies and kittens learn the veterinary hospital is nothing to fear, and a source of pleasant experiences, make a plan for puppies and kittens with behavioral wellness at the core.

To make sure each puppy and kitten gets the care he or she deserves, and each client receives the proper information, schedule extra time for new puppies and kittens. During the initial visits, the technician should take time during the history to assess what treats, toys, and other forms of possible reinforcement the puppy or kitten prefers, and note these in the record. If the patient is wary or fearful during greetings or vital signs, this should also be noted. Worry in puppies and kittens is a sign the animal may be at risk for developing worsening fear, both in the veterinary clinic and at home. Each time the patient is handled by a technician or the veterinarian, the handling should predict the animal's preferred treats, toys, or other rewards to assist in building a positive classically conditioned emotional response to veterinary care. If a puppy or kitten is too stressed to eat or engage in play in the veterinary clinic, it may be necessary to intervene with the more advanced training techniques discussed in subsequent chapters.

Unwanted behaviors are a common cause of animal relinquishment. Preventing unwanted behaviors at home protects pets and preserves the **human–animal bond**, and it keeps pets coming to the veterinary hospital. Discuss normal puppy and kitten behaviors with pet owners during their juvenile wellness visits. Technicians are the perfect people to have these educational talks with pet owners, and because we see puppies and kittens several times during their youth visits, we can break up the information into smaller segments for faster visits and to avoid overwhelming pet owners with too much information at once. Table 4.4 shows the behavior topics we suggest discussing during puppy wellness visits, and Table 4.5 shows the checklist for kitten wellness visits.

Some of the topics included in the wellness checklist include handling exercises. During the wellness visits, the veterinary team should examine the animal, and also teach the owner how to handle the animal. Teach the pet owner exercises such as brushing the teeth, trimming nails, cleaning and inspecting ears, and tolerating light stabilizing restraint using distractions, desensitization, and classical conditioning. At each visit, provide the client with some handling homework to practice between visits. When the puppy or kitten learns to enjoy body handling and husbandry at home with the owner, veterinary care becomes simpler in the clinic, and necessary treatments later in life are much better tolerated at home.

The most common problem home behavior described for both dogs and cats is house soiling.[3] Table 4.6 shows the most common behavior problems that owners describe when surrendering dogs to the shelter; Table 4.7 shows the same for cats. Providing owners with a guide for proper housetraining for puppies and kittens will help the owner have realistic expectations and better success during the housetraining process, preventing unwanted house soiling later in life. Other problem behaviors include destructive behavior, and aggressive behavior toward the owner.[3] Destructive behavior can be normal for both puppies and kittens, but it also can be an indicator of a behavioral disorder. Learn the difference between normal and abnormal behavior, and familiarize yourself with local referral options for behavior disorders if your veterinarian does

Table 4.4 Puppy wellness visit discussion topics.

Age	Discussion topics
8–12 weeks	Enjoying the veterinary clinic
	Puppy biting and appropriate play
	Housetraining
	Crate training
	Positive socialization
	Fear periods and normal development
	Environments
	Surfaces
	People (gender, age, size, voice, and clothing)
	Friendly puppies
	Gentle adult dogs
	Other animals
	Leashes, harnesses, and collars
	Choosing a puppy class
12–16 weeks	Puppy biting and appropriate play
	Chewing, teething, and appropriate chew items
	Housetraining check-in
	Preventing boredom
	Appropriate physical exercise
	Appropriate mental exercise
	Positive socialization check-in
	Voluntary veterinary home care
	Restraint acceptance
	Home physical exam
	Ear care
	Eye care
	Toothbrushing
	Voluntary grooming
	Nail care
	Coat care
	Choosing an adolescent dog class
16+ weeks	Housetraining check-in
	Appropriate play check-in
	Normal adolescent behavior
	Verify adolescent dog class selected

not offer behavioral therapies. Aggression toward people can include normal jumping, vigorous play, mouthing during play, clawing at the owner during play, grabbing clothing, stalking and ambushing, and more. Each of these are normal behaviors for puppies and kittens, and the owner should be advised to use positive reinforcement and negative punishment to help puppies and kittens learn appropriate forms of play and interaction. Positive punishment is not appropriate.

Table 4.5 Kitten wellness visit discussion topics.

Age	Discussion topics
8–12 weeks	Enjoying the veterinary clinic
	Stalking, biting, and appropriate play
	Litter training
	Carrier training
	Choosing a scratching post/tree
	Scratching post training
	Positive socialization
	Environments
	Surfaces
	People (gender, age, size, voice, and clothing)
	Other animals
	Attending kitten classes where available
12–16 weeks	Appropriate play check-in
	Litter training check-in
	Enrichment for indoor cats
	Preventing boredom
	Appropriate physical exercise
	Appropriate mental exercise
	Positive socialization check-in
	Voluntary veterinary home care
	Restraint acceptance
	Home physical exam
	Ear care
	Eye care
	Toothbrushing
	Voluntary grooming
	Nail care
	Coat care
16+ weeks	Litter training check-in
	Appropriate play check-in
	Destructive behavior Q & A

A good training class will cover all of these common topics, and help support owners during what can be a challenging developmental period for both puppies and kittens.[4, 5] Choosing to provide puppy and kitten classes is a good way for clinics to assure these owners are receiving the best information (Figure 4.9). Attending positive reinforcement classes has the bonus benefit of teaching puppies and kittens to love visiting the hospital. If offering classes isn't a good fit for an individual practice, referral information for appropriate classes should be provided during the first puppy or kitten checkup. Team members should visit a class prior to referring clients, to assure the class is using recommended methods and techniques. Puppies and kittens can attend classes starting

Table 4.6 Most common unwanted behaviors according to owners surrendering dogs to the animal shelter.

Owner-defined behavior problem	Prevalence (%)
House soiling	18.5
Destructive outside	12.6
Aggressive toward people	12.1
Escapes	11.6
Too active	11.4
Needs too much attention	10.9
Vocalizes too much	10.7
Bites	9.7
Destructive indoors	9.7
Disobedient	9

Table 4.7 Most common unwanted behaviors according to owners surrendering cats to the animal shelter.

Owner-defined behavior problem	Prevalence (%)
House soiling	37.7
Destructive indoors	11.4
Aggressive toward people	10.9
Doesn't get along with other pets	8
Bites	8
Needs too much attention	6.9
Unfriendly	6.9
Destructive outdoors	5.1
Requested behavior euthanasia	4.6
Too active	4.6

at eight weeks of age, as long as the classes are structured to be safe and appropriate for that age group. The ideal window of opportunity for socialization closes by 16 weeks for these young animals, so earlier is best when starting classes.

4.4 Hospitalization, Treatments, Diagnostics, and Boarding

Moving through the hospital or having to stay in the hospital can be stressful for both the pet and the client. The same principles of preparing the animal areas to be patient-friendly, and using techniques that are sensitive to the behavioral needs of the patient, apply in the back of the hospital just as they do in the examination room.

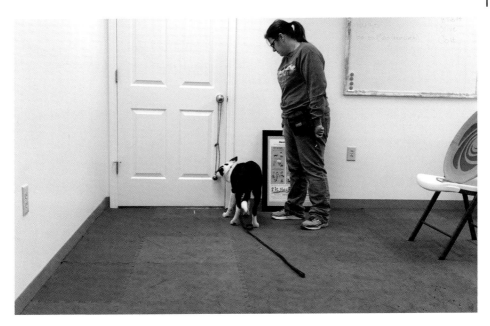

Figure 4.9 Puppy classes help build skills such as housetraining to set up patients for success.

Hospitalization

When possible, hospitalized or boarding patients should be separated by species. If your hospital does not have enough space for separate dog and cat wards, at least keep the species as far apart as possible, and provide visual barriers so they do not have to see one another. Alicea's hospital, Hillview, sees dogs, cats, exotics, and wildlife. Alicea brought her small terrier to the clinic one day, and she was housed in the dog ward while her owner was attending to other patients. In a few hours, Alicea checked on her terrier during a break and found someone had kenneled a goose nearby. The goose seemed comfortable, but the terrier was very excitable and stressed by the presence of the goose. Her panting, pacing, and excitement resulted in her developing hyperthermia at 105.6 °F. Harmful experiences in the wards are not restricted to fear: even too much excitement can be harmful to patients in the hospital.

Patient Movements

Moving patients through the hospital in a thoughtful way reduces stress. The foundation behavior of targeting helps simplify patient movements. The handler should face the direction they want the dog to travel, and encourage using a target or lure as needed. Using a long spoon with sticky food as a lure for animals who haven't learned targeting is often effective. Remember: the lure needs to be achievable, and the dog allowed to eat a bit every few steps so he keeps moving. Make sure the route is clear before moving through, so the dog is protected from interactions with other patients. There should be a relaxed "U" in the leash between the handler and the dog whenever possible. If the dog is very reluctant to move, invite the owner to come with you during the movement, as many dogs will move better with the owner. Make sure dogs learn that moving into and through the hospital is pleasant, and changes in the environment predict high-value rewards.

For example:

- Dog exits vehicle (change in environment) → 3 treats delivered
- Dog walks through parking lot → Treats delivered approximately every 10 feet
- Dog walks through entrance → 3 treats delivered
- Dog walks through reception area → Treat delivered
- Dog approaches treatment room door → Place 4–6 treats on the floor and let the dog eat them while the door is opened
- Dog moves through treatment room door → Toss 4–6 treats on the floor and allow the dog to eat them while the owner moves back to the reception area.

Figure 4.10 diagrams the use of different treat quantities during a dog's journey through the hospital.

The same target or lure can be used to encourage the dog to enter a kennel. Set up any items in the kennel first, such as bedding and water. Encourage the dog to enter the kennel by facing the direction you want him to go, placing the target or lure of a few treats inside the kennel, and then stepping behind the dog to discourage backward movement. In some cases, you may have to gently lift the dog. Do not drag the dog, or lift him and let him drop onto the floor of the kennel, as this will only increase his fear and make him more difficult to kennel in the future.

When removing a shy dog from the kennel, approach the kennel with a leash and treats. Stand with your side or back to the door, and crack the door while offering treats at the level of the leash. Control the door with your body to prevent escape, and allow the dog to come to you. If the dog has a good target behavior, using a hand target or spoon will encourage him to come to you and allow leash placement.

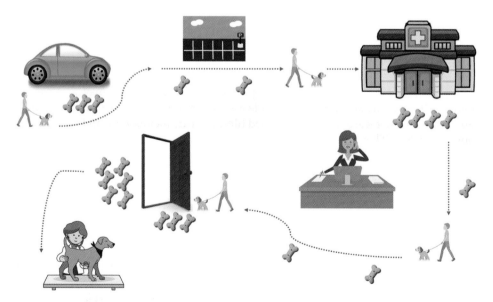

Figure 4.10 Treat flowchart. Each major change in the environment, such as going through a door or into a new room, should predict several treats. Placing several treats on the floor while the dog approaches the door of the exam room, and then 4–6 treats on the floor inside the exam room, will help create a positive emotional response.

If the dog is overly friendly or anxious and bouncing at the door of the kennel, toss a few treats to the back of the kennel so the dog moves away long enough for you to undo the latch and control the door with your body. Offer treats at nose level to encourage him to place his head through the leash, then open the door and allow him to join you outside the kennel.

Video 4.7 shows an excited French bulldog, Ollie. He leaps out of the cage to greet every team member with joy. Sara uses treats in her right hand to feed Ollie as she slips the leash over with her left hand. Notice she placed the leash around her right arm so that the puppy can keep eating the treats without interruption while she loops his leash on. Sara also uses food lures to get him to follow her. To return this excited puppy back to his kennel, Sara uses tiny treats to lure him toward and then into the kennel.

Moving cats should use the same low-stress principles, but the techniques are different since cats will sometimes be transported in a carrier rather than on a leash. When using a carrier, hold the carrier from the bottom rather than the handle for added stability, and cover the carrier with a pheromone-treated towel to avoid the cat seeing people or other animals during transport. Some cats are more comfortable being carried in a towel while eating treats. Choose the method that helps the cat remain the most relaxed, and always check your route in advance to assure you won't be surprised by passing other animals. Verify the ward cage or kennel is set up with any bedding, litter, and water in advance, leaving enough room for the carrier to fit inside the kennel. Place the carrier inside the kennel, and open the door, allowing the cat to come out at his own pace. Once the cat has come out of the carrier, remove the carrier.

Some shy cats will not come out of the carrier on their own when people are around. For these cats, remove the door of the carrier but leave the box itself in the kennel to provide a safe hiding area. When the cat needs to be treated, use the carrier to transport the cat out of the kennel, and gently disassemble the carrier around the cat if more access is needed. Avoid pulling or dumping the cat out of the carrier.

Dog Wards

Mitigating sound is important in dog wards. Preventing stress can help reduce barking. Also, housing barking dogs in a separate, quiet area, if one is available, may decrease the domino effect of one dog initiating a whole ward of barking. If possible, provide sound-reducing acoustic measures such as baffled tiles, acoustic membranes, and an acoustic-muffling ceiling. There are many noise-reducing building materials available, and these can help both dogs and humans have a better quality of life in the dog ward.

Provide acoustic therapy such as music ("Through a Dog's Ear," for example). Pheromone diffusers should be used in the ward, and when possible the bedding can also be treated with pheromones. If possible, the owner can provide bedding such as a towel or familiar mat from home as well as the dog's favorite treats. A nonslip mat or yoga mat should be placed under any slick bedding to prevent the animal from sliding around. Caution pet owners that the mat or bed might become soiled, so they select an appropriate item. Visual barriers across part of the door of the kennel can be helpful for shy or nervous dogs, so they do not see and interact with passing patients. Blankets and towels make good impromptu barriers. Corrugated plastic boards (this looks like corrugated cardboard, but it is constructed from lightweight plastic) can also be cut to fit the fronts of cage doors and affixed to the outside of the door. This plastic can be fully disinfected and used many times before it wears out. For sliding glass doors, an inexpensive privacy film can be applied to the bottom half of the door so that people passing by can easily check on the well-being of the patient, but dogs walking by will not be visible. Food and treats can be provided in a puzzle toy or food dispenser (Figure 4.11). Choose food toys and dispensers that can be easily washed and disinfected. If the dog is

(a)

(b)

(c)

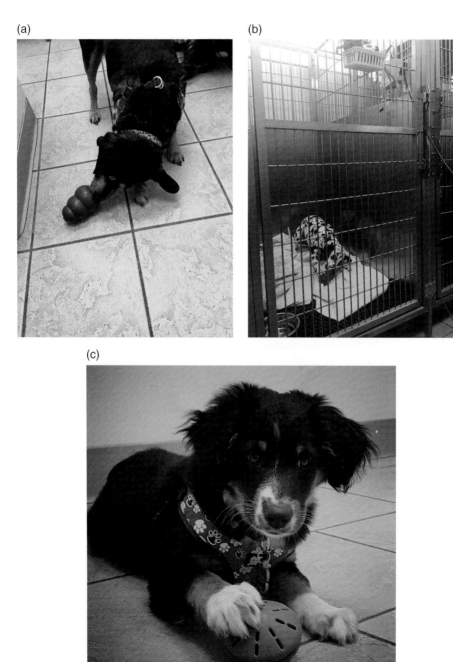

Figure 4.11 (a–c) Dogs using food toys in the hospital.

not accustomed to using a food-dispensing toy, make sure to record food intake in the record and provide food in a dish if the dog is not using the toy.

Cat Wards

Most cats love having a place to hide while they are in the wards. A carrier without a door can be provided, but a cardboard box, reusable cots covered in a towel, fancy cat condos, or even paper shopping sacks will do. There are commercially available cat ward boxes that provide a place for litter, an enclosed hiding area, and an elevated resting platform (Figure 4.12). A towel or corrugated plastic barrier can be placed over at least half of the cage door so the cat can choose to be visible or hidden, but the team can easily check on the cat at any time (Figure 4.13). Encourage cat owners to bring a towel, mat, or small bed from home that is familiar to the cat, but do caution the owner that the item may become soiled. Pheromone diffusers should be plugged in around the ward, and bedding as well as cage door covers can be treated with pheromones as well.

Instruct cat owners to bring their favorite food and treats from home, and ask what kind of litter the cat prefers. If the litter type is unusual, it is best for the owner to provide litter as well. Most cats prefer unscented, fine-grit litter.[6] Choose a litter of this type for your daily in-hospital use.

Treatment Rooms

If the authors had a magical low-stress genie in a lamp granting three wishes, here are our wishes:

1) Every pet arrives hungry and with his favorite treats from home.
2) No-restraint and low-restraint care become standard operating procedures.
3) Stop taking animals away from their owners, or "to the back" for treatments that can easily be performed in an exam room.

Taking animals to the treatment room without the owner can cause unnecessary stress for both the patient and the client. While some animals may seem "better without the owner," this effect is generally caused by learned helplessness rather than true comfort. Does the animal accept treats in the same fashion, have more loose and happy body language, and choose to be closer to the veterinary team in the treatment room? Use the patient assessment tools to determine if an animal is truly "better" without the owner.

The authors understand that some team members are uncomfortable working in front of the owner. We are both full-time technicians in private practice, and we used to be nervous about it, too! With regular practice, this feels normal to team members, confidence grows, and the clients are amazed at what we can accomplish. We also understand that some owners may contribute negatively to the patient experience by talking loudly, scolding the animal, or trying rough restraint. Most owners are simply nervous or embarrassed themselves, and will respond well to good instructions from you. Coaching the owner on how to talk to the patient, where to stand, and how to give food will help calm the situation. For example, if the owner is nervous, noisy, and touching the animal inappropriately, I may provide the owner with 20 tiny treats and instruct her to deliver one treat per second. Both of her hands will be occupied by the treat-counting task, and her voice will be calmer and counting rather than anxious. If the owner strongly prefers not to

(a)

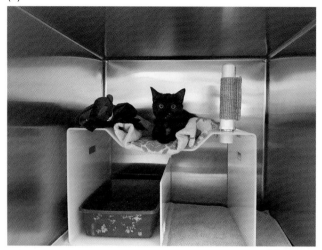

(b)

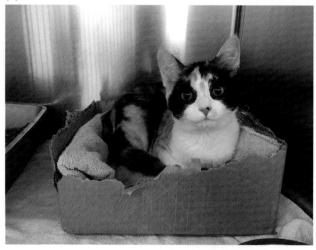

Figure 4.12 Examples of hiding places for cats in the hospital.

be present for injections, nail trims, anal gland expression, blood collection, subcutaneous fluids, or the many other simple procedures performed in the exam room, simply have the owner step into the lobby rather than moving the patient.

When it is necessary to move a patient to the treatment room, check to make sure the treatment area is available, and there are no other patients nearby. Set up everything needed for the procedure prior to moving the patient, including a hospital cage for when you've completed the procedure if you're hospitalizing the patient. Communicate with team members so they know you'll be working in the treatment room, and not to show up with a barking terrier while you're placing an IV catheter in an anxious cat. When moving through the treatment area, prevent social interactions between patients (Figure 4.14). Table 4.8 is a checklist to guide procedural setup prior to moving the patient.

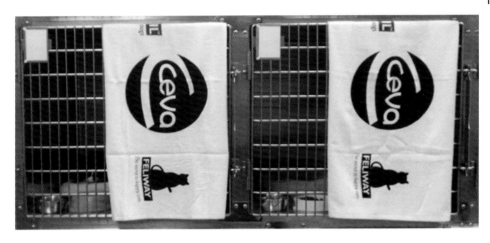

Figure 4.13 Partially covering the door of a kennel gives the cat an option to hide while allowing the team to check on the cat as well.

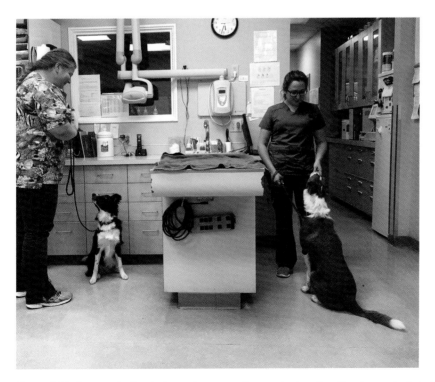

Figure 4.14 Communication between team members and using visual barriers protects patients from social interactions in the treatment room.

Table 4.8 Checklist for procedures outside the exam room.

Procedure checklist
☐ Plan where to perform procedure.
☐ Recon the route: check for other patients before moving.
☐ Set up the destination area before moving (patient entered in computer for x-rays, ultrasound machine set up for cystocentesis, etc.).
☐ Explain procedure to client before moving patient.
☐ Invite patient to procedure area using luring, targeting, etc.
☐ Perform procedure as promptly as possible.
☐ Return patient to client or to ward as appropriate.

Minimize noise levels in the treatment room, such as boisterous laughter and rapid movements. Keep music levels low, and be considerate with use of equipment such as dental scalers, compressors, vacuum cleaners, suction pumps, and such. These activities can contribute to trigger stacking for patients who are waiting or being treated in the treatment room.

Radiology

Radiology is a ward where some manual restraint is usually required unless patients are sedated. Sedating stable patients for radiographs will reduce stress and anxiety, improve the quality of films, decrease the number of reshoots needed, decrease the number of staff members in the room during radiograph exposure, and minimize exposure of the team to scatter radiation. We advocate sedation for radiographs whenever possible for all of these reasons (some states require sedation for all radiographs; check your practice act). Painful animals should always receive analgesia prior to radiography, unless the situation is critical and analgesia would present life-threatening complications.

Prior to taking the patient to radiology, make sure the machine and table are fully set up. Input the animal into the computer or make the flash ID card, set the technique, and gather any positioning devices you may need such as a soft V-tray or foam positioning cushions, as well as any treats or distractions to be used (Figure 4.15). Collimate the beam, and position the tube head properly. If you're using a film cassette in the tabletop technique, be sure to place a nonslip mat on the table so both the cassette and the patient will be stable and not move. Dress in your gown, other personal protective equipment, and badge if you'll be in the room during the radiograph, then move the patient into the radiology ward.

Many pets will be frightened by noises in radiography such as moving the tube head, activating the rotor with the pedal, and even the swoosh of Velcro® letting go when we remove gowns. Plan to use masking noises and treats during those times to help dogs relax. Use something soft and sticky for healthy pets for getting onto the x-ray table, sitting, lying down, and curling onto a side (Figure 4.16). If you're not sure if the dog will cooperate for positioning, do a luring dry run in the exam room with the owner, and make the client a part of the anxiolytic/sedation decision-making process prior to taking the animal to radiology. Cats will sometimes eat on the x-ray table, and can be positioned and then immediately returned to eating.

(a)   (b)

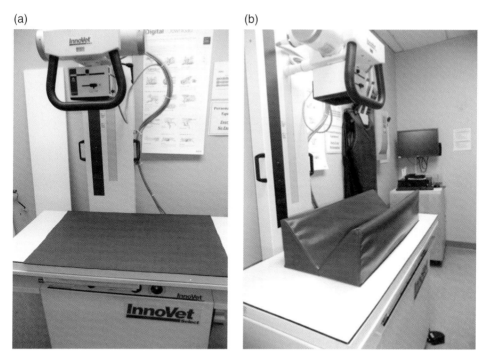

Figure 4.15 (a–b) Using nonslip surfaces and soft positioning aids increases patient comfort in radiology.

Patients who are too sick to eat are often debilitated and easier to handle. Remember to monitor these patients for signs of stress and fear; struggling is not the only way these patients communicate with us. Keep procedures brief, use modified positioning when necessary, and communicate with the team and attending veterinarian if there are problems with obtaining radiographs.

Video 4.8 demonstrates radiographic positioning and decision making. Part 1 shows a mock-up of radiograph positioning for a Golden retriever puppy who had eaten a piece of tennis ball. By smearing peanut butter on the table, the veterinary team is able to encourage the puppy to cooperate for positioning for a lateral radiograph. (Gloves are not worn in the video because it is for training practice, and no exposure was performed.)

Part 2 shows the same dog, now an adolescent who had consumed a piece of hard dog toy, and the veterinarian ordered a survey radiograph. The dog seemed comfortable on the table, but became very fearful when lateral recumbency was attempted. The technician notified the veterinarian, and a dorsoventral view was authorized as an alternative. The technician then worked with the dog to get him more comfortable on the table in sternal recumbency so the dorsoventral view could be performed. After the radiograph, the dog was treated for his gastrointestinal (GI) upset, but also signed up for happy visits and sent home with handling homework so his future veterinary care will be less stressful.

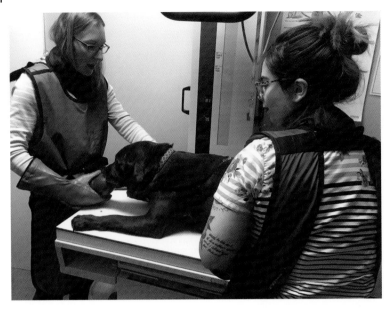

Figure 4.16 Sticky treats delivered in a food toy help this excited patient cooperate for radiographs.

Anesthesia and Surgery

Surgical patients need to be **NPO**.... Or do they? Some anesthesia studies in both pets and people suggest a small amount of food before surgery is beneficial, particularly for diabetic and pediatric patients, or those with very small body mass.[7, 8] That being said, giving water-consistency food such as broth, watered-down baby food, or watered-down canned pet food (either frozen or at room temperature) is a good way to give premedication and collect preoperative lab samples. In general, we suggest collecting preoperative lab work a few days prior to the procedure so that any abnormalities can be addressed without the animal spending excess time in the hospital, and so the blood collection appointment is brief and pleasant for the patient; but sometimes this is not possible based on the patient, the clinic's policies, or the workflow of the hospital.

Pre-anesthesia medications reduce anxiety, provide preemptive analgesia, decrease the volume of induction agent required, and decrease the amount of volatile anesthetic required. Pre-anesthesia medications should be considered for every anesthesia patient.[9] After pre-anesthesia medications have been given, intravenous (IV) access can be comfortably established in the vast majority of patients (>95% in the authors' combined experience). For dogs who are very nervous even after the premedication, there are several options. Adding to the premedication, placing a standing lateral saphenous catheter, or giving the induction agent using a butterfly catheter in the lateral saphenous so that anesthesia and IV access can be established are all options. Using a topical anesthetic cream at the site of IV access can help make the process more comfortable. Remember: increased stress levels prior to anesthesia are correlated with increased anesthesia complications. Reducing stress before anesthesia is associated with better outcomes.[9] For cats who are still anxious after the pre-anesthesia medications, consider giving additional premedication, and using a gentle towel wrap and giving the induction agent with a butterfly in the medial saphenous vein, then intubating and establishing IV access.

Recovery can be a stressful time for animals as well. Assure the animal has a comfortable place to recover, and a dedicated technician during the recovery process. The animal should be gently supported as needed, and if the patient is experiencing significant dysphoria, medical management for dysphoria is appropriate. Postoperative dysphoria represents considerable distress, and should be treated as such.

Patients who have increased anxiety in the veterinary hospital should receive pre-visit medications at home prior to the surgery appointment, and be first in line for surgery to minimize wait times. When possible, schedule the admission appointment so the owner can be with the patient during the pre-anesthetic medication administration. While the patient is in the hospital, try to have one team member be that patient's "person" for the day to offer continuity and predictability. Lastly, schedule a discharge appointment as early in the day as possible; or, for some patients, having the owner be present during the recovery process is best for everyone involved.

References

1 Volk, J., *et al.* (2011) Executive summary of the Bayer veterinary care usage study. *Journal of the American Veterinary Medical Association.* 238 (10), 1275–1282. https://doi.org/10.2460/javma.238.10.1275

2 Crowell-Davis, S., *et al.* (2004) Social organization in the cat: A modern understanding. *Journal of Feline Medicine and Surgery.* 6 (1), 19–28. http://journals.sagepub.com/doi/abs/10.1016/j.jfms.2003.09.013

3 Salman, M., *et al.* (2000) Behavioral reasons for relinquishment of dogs and cats to 12 shelters. *Journal of Applied Animal Welfare Science.* 3 (2), 93–106. https://doi.org/10.1207/S15327604JAWS0302_2

4 Shaw, K., and Martin, D. (2015) *Canine and Feline Behavior for Veterinary Technicians and Nurses.* Ames, IA: John Wiley & Sons.

5 Overall, K. (2013) *Manual of Clinical Behavioral Medicine for Dogs and Cats.* St. Louis, MO: Mosby.

6 Neilson, J. (2004) Thinking outside the box: Feline elimination. *Journal of Feline Medicine and Surgery.* 6(1), 5–11. https://doi.org/10.1016/j.jfms.2003.09.008

7 Looney, A. (2008) The association of shelter veterinarians veterinary medical care guidelines for spay-neuter programs. *Journal of the American Veterinary Medical Association.* 233(1), 74–86.

8 Manchikanti, L. (2011) Preoperative fasting before interventional techniques: Is it necessary or evidence-based? *Pain Physician.* 14, 459–467.

9 Muir, W. (2013) *Handbook of Veterinary Anesthesia.* St. Louis, MO: Elsevier.

5

Level One Patients and Training

5.1   Introduction to the Levels of Training

Different patients have different needs, and will benefit from individualized training programs. Now that you understand the importance of a clinic culture embracing stress reduction, how animals sense and perceive the environment, how to set up the environment for success, how animals learn, and what the foundation needs are for both trainers and patients, you're ready to start training.

Animals fear veterinary care for a variety of reasons: lack of positive emotional conditioning, negative learning experiences in the past, genetics, socialization, and more. The animal's stress level will dictate which methods are most appropriate to start out. The goal of any training plan is to reduce stress and anxiety, increase compliance, and improve the veterinary experience for the patient, client, and veterinary team. Most animals will respond to training, and will have noticeably decreased stress levels. However, some patients may not progress as we hope. Some animals appear stressed both at home and in the hospital, while others relax more easily. Selecting an appropriate training plan, setting realistic expectations, and adapting to the animal in front of you will improve outcomes.

This guide uses patient assessments to divide patients into three categories: Level One, Level Two, and Level Three. Each level has a tailored training plan template based on that group's stress level and specific needs (Figure 5.1). We will use the same assessment tool introduced in earlier chapters:

1) Food acceptance, toy acceptance, and tactile acceptance
2) Body language
3) Proximity preference.

5.2   Identifying Level One Patients

When assessing patients, it is important to remember that every animal makes decisions, thinks, and changes over time. These changes can be moment-to-moment, or visit-to-visit. Each assessment is a snapshot of an instant in time, and veterinary team members need to be fluid and flexible, changing plans and expectations if the

Cooperative Veterinary Care, First Edition. Alicea Howell and Monique Feyrecilde.
© 2018 John Wiley & Sons, Inc. Published 2018 by John Wiley & Sons, Inc.
Companion website: www.wiley.com/go/howell/cooperative

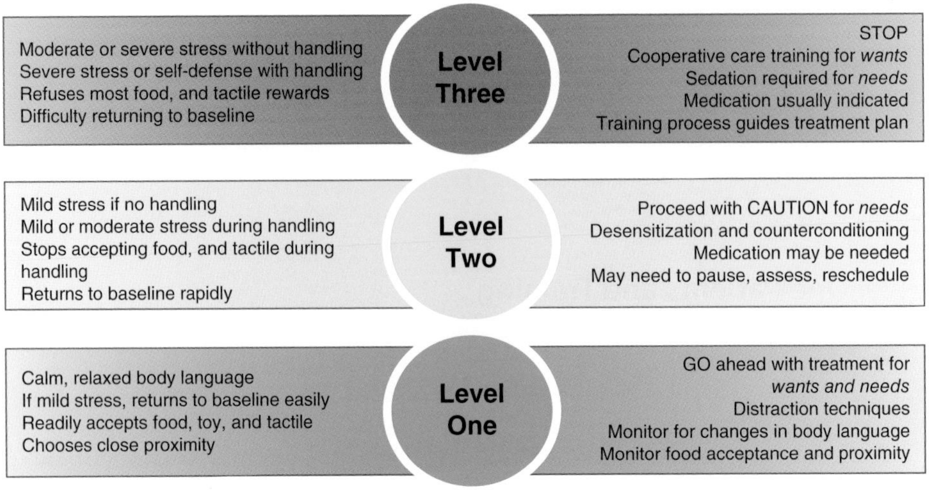

Moderate or severe stress without handling Severe stress or self-defense with handling Refuses most food, and tactile rewards Difficulty returning to baseline	**Level Three**	STOP Cooperative care training for *wants* Sedation required for *needs* Medication usually indicated Training process guides treatment plan
Mild stress if no handling Mild or moderate stress during handling Stops accepting food, and tactile during handling Returns to baseline rapidly	**Level Two**	Proceed with CAUTION for *needs* Desensitization and counterconditioning Medication may be needed May need to pause, assess, reschedule
Calm, relaxed body language If mild stress, returns to baseline easily Readily accepts food, toy, and tactile Chooses close proximity	**Level One**	GO ahead with treatment for *wants and needs* Distraction techniques Monitor for changes in body language Monitor food acceptance and proximity

Figure 5.1 The levels of training. Level One, Level Two, and Level Three patients will each be assessed and identified, and appropriate training techniques selected.

Table 5.1 Checklist for Level One dogs: Each dog assessing at Level One should have each of these attributes.

Stage of visit	Food acceptance	Body language	Proximity preference
Greeting	☐ From any team member ☐ Within 5 seconds ☐ Soft mouth	☐ Relaxed body	☐ Greets immediately ☐ Stays near team member ☐ Solicits attention
Touching	☐ From any team member ☐ Soft mouth ☐ Throughout touching	☐ Relaxed during touch	☐ Does not move away ☐ Remains close when touched
Exam & treatment	☐ From any team member ☐ Soft mouth ☐ Throughout procedures	☐ Relaxed during handling	☐ Does not move away ☐ Remains close during treatments

patient's status changes. Level One patients are relaxed or experiencing minimal stress. Table 5.1 provides a checklist to assist with this assessment. Figure 5.2 shows images of a Level One dog.

Level One Dogs

Food Acceptance
- Dogs will accept food immediately or after <5 seconds
- Will accept food from any team member

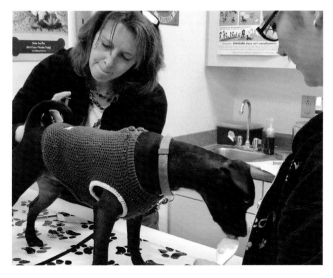

Figure 5.2 Level One canine patient.

- Takes food with a soft mouth; no snapping or grabbing
- Continues accepting food even when touched
- Accepts food before, during, and after procedures

Body Language
- Relaxed body language (refer to Chapter 2)
- Remains relaxed during touching and handling
- Remains relaxed during procedures

Proximity Preference
- On-leash and off-leash, dog immediately greets veterinary team members
- Chooses to remain near team members while they talk to and touch him
- Does not back away or move away when approached
- Does not back away or move away when touched
- Remains near team members during procedures

Level One Cats

Food acceptance is a less reliable indicator of stress in cats when contrasted against dogs. Many dogs will accept food when stressed, and many cats will refuse a variety of food treats even when they are calm and comfortable at home. However, for cats who will eat in the hospital, changes in food acceptance are a useful indicator of stress levels. In general, kittens who learn to enjoy food treats in the hospital will continue to do so as adults. Many kittens and adult cats will also interact with a toy even if they aren't interested in food, so toy acceptance is also included in the feline assessment. Table 5.2 is a checklist to assist in assessing Level One feline patients. Figure 5.3 shows a Level One cat.

Table 5.2 Checklist for Level One cats: Each cat assessing at Level One should have each of these attributes.

Stage of visit	Food acceptance	Body language	Proximity preference
Greeting	☐ From any team member ☐ Shows strong interest ☐ May eat within 30 seconds ☐ May prefer toy ☐ May prefer tactile	☐ Relaxed body	☐ Exits carrier willingly ☐ Explores exam room ☐ Solicits attention
Touching	☐ From any team member ☐ Not diminished by touch	☐ Relaxed during touch	☐ Does not move away ☐ Remains close when touched
Exam & treatment	☐ From any team member ☐ Not diminished by procedure	☐ Relaxed during handling	☐ Does not move away ☐ Remains close during treatments

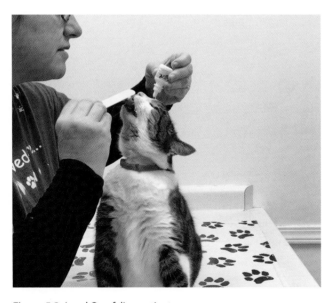

Figure 5.3 Level One feline patient.

Food Acceptance, Toy Acceptance, and Tactile Acceptance
- Accepts food while in carrier, or within 30 seconds of exiting carrier
- Interacts with toy if toy motivated
- Investigates offered food, but may or may not eat depending upon preferences
- Accepts food before, during, and after touching
- Accepts food before, sometimes during, and after procedures
- Accepts tactile rewards before, sometimes during, and after procedures

Body Language
- Relaxed body language (refer to Chapter 2)
- Remains relaxed during touching and handling
- Remains relaxed before, during, and after procedures

Proximity Preference
- Chooses to exit carrier
- Explores exam room willingly
- Approaches team members within 30 seconds of exiting carrier
- Will rub against team members' legs
- Will head bump and allow touching and facial rubbing
- Remains near team members during touching and handling
- Remains near team members before, during, and after procedures

Patients who are appropriate for Level One training are largely comfortable with the environment and procedures from the start. Level One training is a combination of distractions, luring, and classical conditioning to maintain this relaxed state (Figure 5.4). Treating fear is much like treating pain: it is far easier to prevent than it is to reverse. By using Level One training techniques for relaxed patients, we teach the patients to remain relaxed and develop positive emotional responses. Level One training should be basic hospital policy for relaxed patients to keep them relaxed in the long term and build a positive and trusting relationship. Rewarding patients for "doing nothing" while they are being treated will teach them how to cooperate for procedures, and how to enjoy veterinary visits.

Individual patients may also assess as different levels based on their health status and the procedures required. For example, some dogs may be Level One dogs for everything except nail trimming, and assess as Level Three when a nail trim is attempted. A normally relaxed cat may assess at Level One for an annual examination

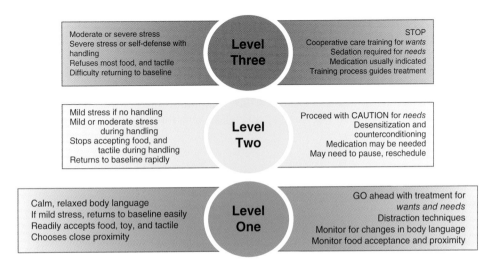

Figure 5.4 Level One patient assessment.

and vaccinations, but as Level Two when she is presented for limping. As always, we must remain flexible during our assessments, and adjust to work with the patient in front of us in real time.

Video 5.1 shows an example of a dog moving from Level One, to Level Two, to Level Three, all in a few short moments. Buster the Pit bull terrier is relaxed and eating the food reinforcement while being examined, which is Level One. During the physical exam, he starts to show some mild to moderate stress markers of avoidance and backing off, especially when touched around his face and ears; this is Level Two. The doctor continues her exam and then injects a vaccine, at which point Buster changes to Level Three. He shows body language consistent with severe stress, including a (fortunately) inhibited bite. This video is a good example of how the levels can change rapidly and of the patient showing conflict behaviors before the snap.

Every interaction is a training opportunity, whether we are choosing to train or not. Understanding classical conditioning, operant conditioning and the value of positive reinforcement, the fundamentals of training, and the foundation behaviors every patient should learn is a great start to making training plans. Training plans need not be complicated, but the more complex the goal behavior, the more complex by necessity the training plan will be.

Making a training plan for any level patient starts with the patient assessment. What is the patient's stress level? Regardless of the level of training needed, the basic flow for creating a training plan will remain the same:

1) Identify the patient's stress level and how it is being measured (panting, lip licking, moving away from the veterinary team, etc.).
2) Identify a nonstressful starting point for training. This includes when, where, who, what, and how much you will train.
3) Identify stopping points in advance. For example: Moving away from the station, avoiding touch, or body language changes.
4) Develop a reinforcement hierarchy. What does the pet prefer, and in what order?
5) Identify the training goal. Determine what method(s) you will use. If DS/CC (desensitizing and counter-conditioning), design the exposure ladder for desensitization. If OC (operant conditioning), make a shaping plan including a variety of approximations to look for.
6) Identify the point of consent. How will the animal tell you he is ready to work?
7) Identify how the animal can withdraw consent, and be ready to stop if they do.
8) Identify the desired cue or cues for the completed behavior.
9) Make a plan for how to fade prompts, lures, and modeling if they will be used.
10) Determine how to introduce duration and release cues for the behavior if appropriate.

5.3 Level One Training: Dog Exam Room and Examination

Remember: every interaction is a training opportunity, because patients are always learning while they are in the hospital. For each training level, we will present common scenarios that veterinary teams encounter in the hospital every day. For each scenario, training suggestions will be provided. Use these training suggestions as a scaffold to build a training plan appropriate for the individual patient. Most patients will respond favorably, but remember to constantly assess and reassess the patient's responses for the comfort and safety of the patient and the veterinary team.

Reception, Weight, and Moving to the Exam Room

Dogs can learn to walk with a team member from the moment we greet them in the reception area. Level One dogs will greet the team member in a relaxed or happy and excited way, and will not move away when greeted. Teaching these dogs to walk with the team member is usually a combination of luring and targeting.

A treat trail is one way to lure a Level One dog to accompany a handler. Place a series of treats on the floor, showing the path the dog should take through the lobby, onto the scale, and into the examination room. Treats need to be close enough together so the dog stays interested, but far enough apart so that the dog is motivated to continue moving. As discussed in Chapter 4, if the lure is too difficult because the treats are too infrequent or too difficult to reach, the animal may lose desire to follow. A sticky spoon is another good luring strategy. Coating a large cooking spoon with sticky treats such as spray cheese, cream cheese, canned food, nut butter, or baby food makes a desirable lure. Hold the spoon at nose level, and allow the dog to take a few licks every few steps as he walks along with the handler.

If the dog stops moving, slow the lure down, try a different kind of lure, or select a different training strategy. Do not drag the dog forward by its leash, as this will increase fear and stress, and decrease trust.

If the dog knows a foundation target behavior such as a nose target to a hand, a body target onto a mat, or a nose target to a spoon or other marker, moving through the hospital becomes simple. Face the direction you want the dog to go, and present your hand or the target item at nose level a few steps ahead of the dog. Allow the dog to touch the target, then reinforce with a click or verbal marker and one small treat. Advanced dogs will be able to travel numerous steps for a single reward, while more novice dogs should only be asked to walk a few steps for each click and treat.

In many cases, the owner can be trained in these methods, and the dog and owner can learn together how to move through the lobby, onto the scale, and into an examination room. Once the dog has entered the exam room, toss five to ten treats onto the floor, spread out around the exam room as a small **jackpot** for going into the room and to encourage exploration.

Video 5.2 demonstrates having a puppy follow a food lure spoon through the lobby, onto the scale, and into the exam room. Notice how the technician makes sure the puppy is willing to follow, keeps the leash loose, faces the direction she wants the puppy to go, and keeps the lure accessible so the puppy is frequently rewarded for following. With practice, this puppy will be able to happily move through the lobby, scale, and exam room taking more and more steps between treats.

The Exam Room

Relaxed dogs will approach the technician during the history. Technicians can multi-task while taking the history and work through greetings and behavioral assessments while asking medical questions. Practice feeding happy dogs for every "hello" they offer. Every time a dog approaches the technician, he should be rewarded with food, so the dog is reinforced for approaching and continues to approach more in the future. When the dog approaches and has received a treat, begin greeting the dog. Some dogs will be comfortable with a face-to-face greeting, but most prefer a 45° angle for greetings (Figure 5.5). Once the dog is comfortable staying nearby during the greeting, reach low between the front legs and stroke or scratch the chest while giving a treat. The dog should respond by leaning into the touch. When you move, you may find the dog moves away for a brief period (<5 seconds for a Level One dog), but he should adjust to your movement and rapidly return to baseline, approaching again for a reward.

Training Tip: Welcome All Greetings!

Every happy greeting, even jumping up with excitement, is welcomed in the veterinary setting. Encourage dogs to keep four paws on the floor by offering treats low or dropping them on the floor, then greeting the dog closer to his level. Never punish dogs for excited greetings, as it can increase stress.

It is important to work where a dog is comfortable during the examination and treatments. In many cases, this will mean working on a nonslip mat on the floor, but in some circumstances the dog will need to be lifted to the table. Just because a dog approaches and is comfortable with touching and petting, this does not mean he will be comfortable with being picked up.

When picking up a large dog, two team members should work together to assure the dog is secure and well-supported, and to distribute the load evenly so team members are not injured while lifting. A third team member or the owner can be offering food

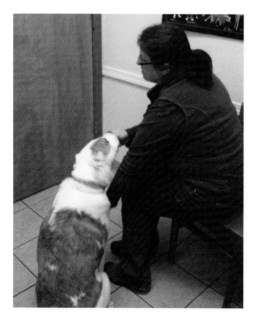

Figure 5.5 Many dogs prefer an angled greeting rather than face-to-face.

while the dog is gently lifted. If the dog stops eating, continue the lift until the dog is safely on the table. If the dog begins to struggle, he is no longer assessing as Level One, and a new plan will be needed.

Video 5.3 shows a team lifting a large dog to the table. The team members do a good job communicating with one another, so the movements are smooth and organized. The dog shows a mild change in her body language when the first technician reaches over her, and when the second technician approaches, but her food acceptance and proximity preference remain at Level One. While the dog is being picked up, she stops eating briefly, but immediately begins eating again once she is on the table. The second time the dog is lifted, her body language is more relaxed, and her food acceptance is improved, evidence that the behavior of allowing lifting is being reinforced. If the dog readily took treats on the floor, but stops accepting treats on the table or tries to escape, she is communicating she is uncomfortable on the table. Try the procedure on the floor instead.

When picking up a small dog, the dog should be well-supported and secure. The technician can squat next to the dog and offer treats, scratching and touching in a similar way as during the greeting. While giving treats with one hand, the technician can stabilize the dog against her leg and hip with the other, then carefully lift the dog onto the table by straightening her legs. In some cases, the dog may be more comfortable being lifted by the owner. The technician should coach the owner on proper lifting technique and assist with treat delivery to assure the dog has a good lifting experience even if the owner is the one doing the lifting. (Some clinics stipulate clients are not allowed to lift animals. Make sure you are familiar with your clinic's policy.)

Video 5.4 shows a small dog approaching the technician and being lifted to the table. The technician assures the dog is securely supported prior to lifting her. She continues to eat treats during the lift and after she is on the table, showing she is comfortable with the lift.

Once the dog is on the table, she should learn the table is a place where good things happen. Frequently deliver small treats or a few licks of a sticky treat throughout the time period the dog is on the table. Giving plenty of small treats will have the effect of classically conditioning the dog to like the table, and operantly conditioning the dog to remain on the table through positive reinforcement. If the dog is taking treats with too much excitement, or is a mouthy puppy, try using a food delivery toy to prolong the treat delivery period and save your hands.

Video 5.5 shows Lloyd having his first blood draw as a puppy. The blood draw is per- formed on the table. The technician verifies Lloyd will take treats on the floor and also on the table, and throughout the blood collection procedure. Lloyd's food acceptance and body language are acceptable throughout the procedure.

Video 5.6 demonstrates the use of a food-dispensing toy on the exam table to encour- age a puppy to enjoy the table and remain relatively still during treatments. The puppy learns the table is a positive place, how to take treats without grabbing hands, and how to remain on the table for treatments.

Physical Examination

In veterinary and technician school, we are taught to perform a physical exam in the same order every time. Having a system is helpful. Systems decrease the chances we will miss something or forget a step. In most cases, we are taught to perform the exam from nose to tail. As discussed in earlier chapters, many patients may find touching of the face and oral cavity stressful, and would prefer not to greet the veterinarian face-to-face. Developing a plan for examining a pet that saves the potentially painful, unpleasant, and socially stressful portions for last will decrease anxiety and increase cooperation. We suggest the following order for physical examination for most patients: general appearance, skin (excluding feet), auscultation, abdominal palpation, lymph nodes, musculoskeletal except paws, neurologic, ears, eyes, oral, paws, rectal/genital. Of course, individual preferences and variations as well as the presenting complaint will modify this order, as they do with any standard examination protocol. Lastly, we should remember wants versus needs. For a healthy patient, the entire exam is a want and can be postponed, modified, or rescheduled when necessary due to patient stress.

During the examination, the patient should always be free to move away if he or she is feeling uncomfortable. The veterinary team will be assessing and reassessing food acceptance, body language, and proximity preference throughout the exam to assure the patient is remaining at Level One.

The technician's role is to provide food treats and keep the veterinarian safe. When giving food, the technician should choose a strategic posture and location where it is easy to observe and assess the animal, and where a bite can be safely prevented if the animal's stress level increases unexpectedly. The technician will also communicate with the veterinarian about changes in food acceptance and body language, alerting the veterinarian to possible increases in anxiety.

Each stage of the examination should predict a small, wonderful food reward. Food should be given freely and frequently enough for the dog to stay interested and cooperative, but rationed in such a way the dog will not become full or satiated prior to completing all the day's procedures.

The skin exam looks like modified petting to the owner, and should feel this way for the dog. As with the greeting, it is usually best to begin by stroking low between the front legs and assessing the patient's response. If the patient remains relaxed, glide the hands over the trunk from ventral to dorsal, examining the skin for abnormalities, masses, and so on. Treats should be given during touching, but withheld between touches. Alternating between examining the skin and giving normal petting will help dogs relax and accept the skin exam as normal.

Auscultation for Level One dogs is generally a smooth process. While maintaining contact from the skin exam, the stethoscope can be removed from the neck, placed in the ears, and introduced to the chest. When changing sides, reach under or over the dog depending on which reach will disturb the dog least. Each of these steps should be paired with a small delicious treat. Some dogs are afraid of the stethoscope and may require Level Two training to accept it.

Palpate the abdomen from beside or behind the dog. When replacing the stethoscope, try to do so with one hand so you can maintain tactile contact without restraining the dog. By maintaining contact, we decrease the effect of startling the dog each time we reestablish contact during the exam. The team member who is feeding and providing stabilization in case of unexpected reactions should also be beside the dog rather than face-to-face with him. The technician who is offering treats and stabilizing the dog should monitor and reassess the patient continuously, alerting the veterinarian or person performing the exam to any changes.

Palpation of the lymph nodes and the musculoskeletal examination can often be combined for good efficiency and to increase patient acceptance. Remaining beside the dog, the veterinarian can palpate the cranial lymph nodes, then the shoulders and neck, prescapular and scapular lymph nodes, then the elbows and forelimb range of motion; and glide down along the spine and ribs, inguinal and popliteal lymph nodes, and then the pelvic limb joints and range of motion. Reflexes such as conscious proprioception may also be appropriate to check at this time.

Once the rest of the body has been examined, it is time to move to more sensitive areas. Some dogs will prefer to look at the veterinarian for the ear, eye, and oral examination, while others will feel more comfortable with the veterinarian approaching from the side. Monitor the patient and select the least stressful approach.

For the ear examination, begin touching in a less sensitive area such as the shoulder or neck, and glide up toward the ear. Inspect the ear visually, and lift the ear flap to examine the pinna and canal. Avoid grasping the pinna by its tip or using the ear as a handle. Throughout this procedure, the technician will be offering small treats. If there is visible inflammation and debris, an otoscope exam may be warranted. Consider placing a topical anesthetic cream on the skin inside of the pinna and vertical canal, then complete the remainder of the physical examination. Placing topical anesthetic will not compromise cytology results and will improve patient comfort during later otoscopic examination. If the ear is infected, Level One training is not appropriate because the patient is in pain.

Targeting or using a food lure can ease examination of the eyes. The technician or veterinarian can help the animal hold still and direct her gaze using treats in different ways: either using a treat spoon to have the animal hold still and the veterinarian moves around to look at the eye, or holding the treat beside your nose to encourage the animal to look at you. Holding a treat near your own nose, and drawing a line between the dog's nose and your own, can help the dog look into your eyes to facilitate examination. Holding a treat beside a light source or ophthalmoscope may help the dog look toward the light source for **PLR** and further ophthalmic evaluation. Cranial nerve responses can also be tested at this time if appropriate for the patient. For tests such as tear tests and corneal staining, Level Two training is usually more appropriate.

Video 5.7 shows the spoon lure technique with Princess Lulu for her physical examination. In Part 5.7b, the cheese keeps a young puppy still enough that the veterinarian can perform an eye examination.

Oral examination for Level One dogs is generally well-accepted. Since the dog has been accepting treats throughout the exam, he has had a chance to become comfortable with fingers and hands near and in his mouth. From one side, lift the lips to see the teeth and gums, and insert a treat. Repeat this process on the opposite side. Stand beside the dog rather than face-to-face when opening the mouth. To open the mouth, use a pretzel rod with a sticky treat, or a sticky treat on your fingers right behind the canines. The dog will generally reach to lick the treats, opening the mouth. You can then gently support the open mouth to see inside.

Some veterinarians like to examine the toenails, toes, and bottoms of the paws with each checkup. Remember that the paws and toes have a high concentration of nerve endings, and are more sensitive to touch. Begin touching in a less sensitive area such as the shoulder or hip, glide a hand down, and gently lift the paw in a normal ergonomic walking position. Monitor the dog for food acceptance and proximity preference.

Many dogs will stop eating while you're touching the foot, but will resume as soon as the foot is put down. If the dog tries to move away or struggle, allow him to move away and reassess the situation to make a new plan.

Last should be the rectal and genital exam. Temperature measurement can be performed at this time, or during the history, depending upon patient preference. To examine the external urogenital and rectal area, begin touching in a less sensitive area such as the shoulder. Glide a hand along the back, and gently displace the tail laterally or lift it. For breeds who carry the tail over the back, Level One dogs have already raised their own tails. For other breeds, avoid raising the tail higher than the level of the spine (parallel with the floor in a standing dog). Excessive elevation of the tail requires a firm grasp and is uncomfortable or painful for some patients. Avoid raising the tail unless it is medically necessary.

5.4   Level One Training: Cat Exam Room and Examination

Level One cats should be comfortable entering and exiting the cat carrier at home and in the veterinary clinic. Pet owners should be instructed in how to condition cats to like the cat carrier rather than take off running as the result of a negative emotional response. Teaching a cat to like her carrier requires a bit of planning combined with a bit of training. First, the carrier should be a normal part of the household furniture at home. The carrier should be placed in an area the cat likes to rest, such as at the base of the cat tree or in a comfortable corner. Place a comfortable bed inside the carrier. The door should be removed or fastened open so the cat does not become accidentally trapped inside. Many cats will choose to rest in the carrier when one is provided as part of the living quarters. Cat owners can place tasty treats inside the carrier, deliver a treat anytime they find the cat resting in the carrier, and place things like catnip inside to encourage the cat to enter and exit the carrier regularly. Cats who understand targeting a spoon or stick will often follow the target into or out of the carrier both at home and in the clinic.

As discussed in Chapter 4, the cat owner should be escorted to the exam room as soon as possible to decrease stressors experienced in the reception area. Carry the kennel from the bottom for a smoother ride. Depending upon patient preference, place the kennel on the floor or an elevated surface in the exam room, opening the door. Allow the cat to acclimate, and offer treats such as canned cat food, cream cheese, butter, fish paste, or cat treats (Figure 5.6). Allow the cat to explore the exam room and approach you to say hello. Every time the cat comes to a veterinary team member, she should be offered a treat, toy play, or pleasurable touch such as stroking the cheeks or chin. Some cats will be more comfortable remaining in the bottom of their carriers (Figure 5.7). Observe the cat during the history and determine which forms of reward the cat prefers, as these will be used during the examination.

Relaxed cats can be lifted gently to the table, assuring they are well-supported. Most cats will not eat while being lifted, but Level One cats will resume interest in treats, toys, or tactile rewards when they are on the table. If the cat chooses not to exit the carrier, the carrier can be placed on the table and the top of the carrier gently removed. As with dogs, the cat should be encouraged to stay on the exam table by the technician who is offering the preferred reward (treats, toys, or tactile) for remaining there. Frequent rewards help to form a positive emotional association with being on the table, and positively reinforce the choice to stay still on the table.

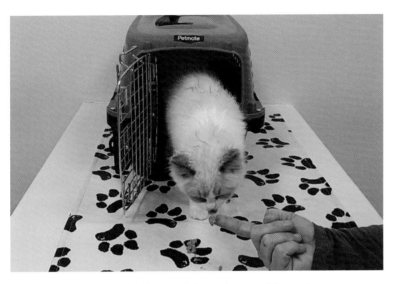

Figure 5.6 Cat following food treats while coming out of the carrier.

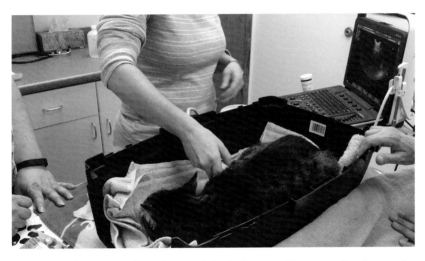

Figure 5.7 Feline patient allowed to remain in the bottom of her carrier for ultrasound.

Physical Examination

The same principles of physical examination for Level One dogs apply for Level One cats. The examination should be performed in order from least invasive to most invasive, saving the oral exam, rectal exam, or any painful areas for last. We need to remember needs versus wants, and that for a healthy cat, a physical examination is a want rather than a need. In some cases, medical management of fear and anxiety is needed, additional training is indicated, and the exam or appointment can be postponed and rescheduled if appropriate.

For physical examination, consider completing the entire examination prior to discussing findings with the owner. Narrate the exam, but avoid pausing for discussion so the examination period is as brief as possible. Most cats also prefer when the veterinarian stands beside rather than face-to-face, as this position is less socially intimidating. When examining the skin, begin by stroking the cheek, chin, and then the neck and shoulders. Begin on the **midline** over the spine, and work downward. Most cats prefer to be touched dorsally rather than ventrally, which is different from dogs. Each touch should predict treats or tactile rewards, which will be given by the technician. The technician should stay ready to provide additional stabilization if the cat has an unexpected reaction, but assessing and monitoring the cat's food acceptance, body language, and proximity preferences will catch stress responses before they manifest as self-defense. For cats, lymph node and thyroid evaluation can be combined with the skin and coat exam.

Next, auscultation should be performed. Stand beside the cat and maintain contact with the cat with one hand while placing the stethoscope in your ears with the other. Introduce the stethoscope dorsally, then slide ventrally to auscult. Cats tend to startle more than dogs when touch is stopped and started, so maintaining contact with at least one hand between touches is often helpful for cats. The technician should be offering preferred rewards throughout this process, and monitoring the cat for changes in food acceptance, body language, and proximity preference.

Abdominal palpation is the next step in the physical examination. Pressure should be applied gradually during palpation, and only to the point where the cat remains comfortable. The technician will continue to provide small treats and tactile rewards during this exam, while being ready to provide stabilization if the cat responds unexpectedly. Abdominal palpation is a good segue into musculoskeletal examination including range of motion of the limbs if indicated, and signs of spinal discomfort.

Saving the most sensitive areas for the end of the exam, the face, feet, and rectogenital examination should be done last. While standing beside the cat, touch is introduced in a less sensitive area such as the shoulder and glides up to the base of the pinna. Many cats have open enough ears so that the pinna does not need to be manipulated. If there is visible otic inflammation or infection, Level Two training and handling will be more appropriate. The eyes can be examined in much the same fashion as for dogs, using a food treat or toy to encourage the cat to gaze in the desired direction. Hold a treat or toy, even something as simple as a moving cotton ball, next to your own temple or nose so the cat will look at you for ocular examination. Level One cats will generally watch this distraction even while an ophthalmoscope or indirect handheld lens is used. More restraint tends to make cats close their eyes or try to escape, compromising the quality of the exam.

Oral examination is crucial for cats whenever possible without causing increased stress levels. Because so many cats (>70% of cats aged 7 and older) have painful tooth resorption, the oral exam should be gentle but thorough.[1] The American Veterinary Dental College states annual dentistry with radiographs is indicated for senior cats even when the visual oral exam is normal because the risk for this silent and painful condition is so high. Stand beside the cat and offer treats if he has been accepting them. Something sticky such as cream cheese or butter is often useful. Offer the treat near the commissure of the lips, then press inward to lift the lip and examine the teeth. Repeat from each side. To open the mouth, use a finger with a treat, or a pretzel rod or tongue depressor with treats, directly behind the canines. Insert the sticky treat, and the cat will generally open. Support the open mouth with your fingers while the cat is licking the food.

Table 5.3 Examination order

Least invasive first: Examination order
General appearance
Skin (excluding feet)
Auscultation
Abdominal palpation
Lymph nodes
Musculoskeletal
Neurologic
Ears
Eyes
Oral
Paws
Rectal/genital
Any known painful areas should be reserved for last

Plan physical examination from least invasive to most invasive, saving any painful areas for the end of the exam. Individual preference may require changes to the examination order, depending upon what a specific patient considers to be invasive.

Video 5.8 shows feline physical and oral examination. Notice the exam is gentle and moves at the pace the cat is comfortable; the use of food encourages him to open his mouth. He stops eating briefly during the middle of the exam, but returns to his treats after the exam is complete.

Lastly, examination of the paws if indicated, and the rectal area. Paw examination is similar to that for dogs. Begin touch in a less sensitive area such as the shoulder or hip near the dorsal midline, then glide down the leg to the paw, lifting the paw in a natural walking posture. To examine the rectal area, begin touching over the shoulder or neck, glide your hand down the dorsal midline, and, using one or two fingers, displace the tail to the side. Rather than grasping the tail, use your fingers in the "OK" sign around the tail to move it aside or minimally lift it. Avoid lifting the tail above the level of the spine, which is parallel with the floor in a standing cat. Many Level One cats will elevate the tail on their own in response to stroking along the spine, or already have the tail elevated when standing simply because they are relaxed, simplifying the genital exam considerably. Table 5.3 summarizes a suggested order for physical examination starting with the probable least stressful portions, and saving the most concerning parts of the exam for last. Individual patient preference will affect the examination order as well.

5.5 Level One Training: Injections and Sample Collection

For Level One animals, the training process is very similar for dogs and for cats for routine procedures. Level One essentially combines luring and distractions with aspects of desensitization to form positive associations with medical procedures, and to decrease the amount of restraint or physical stabilization required to accomplish the procedure.

Subcutaneous and Intramuscular Injection

Subcutaneous injection is the most common route used for injectable agents in small-animal medicine. Both dogs and cats will often remain stationary and cooperative for subcutaneous injection when a distraction such as food treats is provided. **Intramuscular** is another route often used for injections in the veterinary hospital, and many animals will allow the distraction method for this injection.

For both dogs and cats, follow the same basic steps. First, determine what treats or distractor the patient prefers. Assure all materials and treats are ready prior to beginning the injection process. To assess the animal's comfort level with the procedure, begin offering the preferred treat, then touch the injection area lightly. Gradually stroke the injection area more firmly, then tent the skin. Pinch lightly, then firmly, with a fingernail. If the animal continues to remain interested in the distraction and does not move away, give the injection. After the injection, remove the food distraction.

Video 5.7 showed using the distraction method during a vaccination for a Level One dog. The technician introduces the food distraction, then takes several seconds to move through the handling leading up to the injection. Since the dog is relaxed and remains interested in the distraction, the injection is administered. The dog continues eating throughout the injection process, and shows relaxed body language.

Video 5.9 shows two Level One kittens being vaccinated. The technician first checks to assure the kittens are interested in the food distraction, which is canned kitten food. She reaches toward the injection site, tents the skin, pinches with her fingers, and then gives the injection. The first kitten never stops eating and seems not to notice the injection process. For the second kitten (a littermate to the first), she is interested in the food distraction throughout the preparation for injecting. When the technician begins the actual injection, the kitten moves away a few inches and stops eating briefly, but the injection is almost completed so the technician floats along with the kitten to finish the vaccination. As soon as the injection is finished, the kitten returns to relaxed body language and eating her treats.

Video 5.10 shows two different adult cats from the same household. These cats are a good example of choosing the right reward for the right patient. The first cat does well for vaccination with food rewards. She eats throughout the procedure. When we offer food for the second cat, he is less interested, but he likes tactile rewards. He remains relaxed for his injection while tactile rewards are given.

Video 5.11 shows Skittles, a black Labrador retriever, receiving an intramuscular injection. The technician lightly stabilizes Skittles while another assistant provides baby food from a syringe. The veterinarian touches the injection area lightly, then pinches it, then administers the injection. Skittles notices the injection (it stings), but returns to eating right away.

Venipuncture

Cephalic

Cephalic venipuncture is common for both dogs and cats. Many dogs and cats will remain stationary for a food distraction during cephalic venipuncture. Some animals may experience increased stress for this procedure if they dislike nail trimming or paw handling, so consider the animal's individual preferences prior to selecting cephalic venipuncture.

To allow cephalic venipuncture, the animal must allow stabilization of the forelimb, occluding or holding off the vein, alcohol or preparation solution applied to the skin, palpation of the vein, and needle puncture, and must remain stationary for long enough for the sample to be collected.

First, verify what treat or distraction method the animal prefers. One technician or assistant will be stabilizing the patient and providing food distractions, while the second collects blood. The technician who is stabilizing will invite the animal to sit close to her, and begin offering treats. If you are stabilizing the patient, place your arm gently between the dog's or cat's head and the person drawing blood to protect against any unexpected reactions to the needle puncture, and provide treats with the opposite hand. Once the patient is stabilized, the person who is feeding will monitor the patient's food acceptance, body language, and proximity preferences.

The person drawing blood will touch the shoulder, then the elbow, and then occlude the vein, or the person who is stabilizing may also occlude the vein depending upon the phlebotomist's preference. Prior to drawing blood, the technician will stroke the limb, gently hold the limb, apply alcohol, pinch the injection area, and then finally perform venipuncture (Figure 5.8). If the patient shows an increase in fear or anxiety, using a different blood collection site or a Level Two training plan may be more appropriate. In some hospitals and with certain patients, practitioners may choose to have the pet owner administer the food distraction during sample collection, but this varies by hospital policy.

Video 5.12 shows a Level One kitten cephalic venipuncture. The assistant who is stabilizing the kitten gets her interested in the canned food on the tongue depressor, then holds the limb at the elbow and occludes the vein. The technician who is drawing blood palpates the vein, places alcohol, tests the venipuncture site, then collects the blood. The kitten remains interested in the food distraction throughout the procedure. Video 5.13 shows this same procedure with an adult cat.

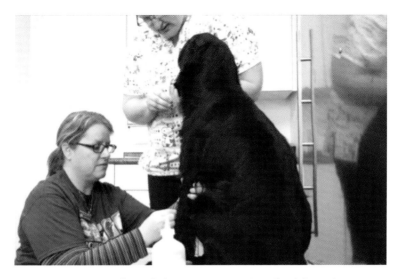

Figure 5.8 Positioning for cephalic venipuncture using a food distraction.

Video 5.14 shows a Level One feline cephalic venipuncture. Everything is going smoothly, but part of the way through the blood collection, the cat has consumed all the food. Observe the cat's body language. It changes rapidly to moderate stress when the food is gone. This error caused the cat to experience more stress than expected during the procedure. Make sure you have plenty of treats at hand before you begin!

Lateral Saphenous (Dogs)

The **lateral saphenous** is an excellent place to collect a sample from a dog who is comfortable standing or lying down on a hip. When collecting from the lateral saphenous, there are several positioning options shown in Figure 5.9. For the three-person option, one person provides treats and stabilizes the dog's front end, while the second occludes the vein and the third draws blood. In the two-person option, the first person provides treats and stabilizes the front of the dog, while the second person both occludes the vessel and collects the blood.

When collecting from the lateral saphenous, remember to have the dog on a comfortable nonslip surface. The dog should be standing or lying down rolled onto a hip. It is not necessary or appropriate to restrain these dogs in lateral recumbency. Offer the treat distraction at nose level, holding it still so the dog remains still. Place an arm near the dog's neck to prevent him from turning around if he is startled by the needle stick. The person who is occluding the vein (whether this is a dedicated team member or the person drawing the blood) should start touch higher on the leg near the hip, then glide down to the back of the stifle to occlude the vessel (Figure 5.10). The person who is offering treats should monitor the dog's body language and food acceptance, and communicate any changes to the rest of the team. Stroke the area where the blood will be drawn, then pinch, apply alcohol, and collect the sample. For patients who tend to move slightly, a butterfly catheter can simplify blood collection as the patient can move a bit and the blood draw can continue.

Medial Saphenous (Cats)

Level One cats will often give blood from the **medial saphenous** while calmly sitting sternal on a table. Please do not scruff and stretch cats for this sample. The cat should be positioned on a comfortable nonslip surface. One person will offer treats and stabilize the cat while occluding the vein, while a second technician collects the blood. Allow the cat to sit in sternal recumbency, rolled onto a hip. While the cat is eating his treats, gently hold off the vein using a few fingers. A whole-hand "karate chop" is not necessary; try to apply the minimum required pressure in the correct location to raise the vein. The person who is stabilizing the cat will monitor body language and food acceptance. When collecting the sample, stroke the sample area, apply alcohol, palpate the vein, pinch to test for reaction, then collect the sample. A butterfly catheter can be very useful in slightly wiggly patients. Video 5.15 demonstrates this technique with a feline patient.

Jugular

The **jugular vein** is a preferred site for venipuncture for rapid blood collection because the sampling time is far shorter, and if the peripheral veins need to be conserved for some reason (e.g., chemotherapy, or an IV catheter anticipated within the next week). If a volume of blood larger than 3 ml is required, the jugular vein will supply this sample size easier than peripheral veins. However, jugular access may be slightly more invasive from the animal's perspective.

(a)

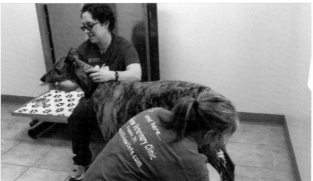

(b)

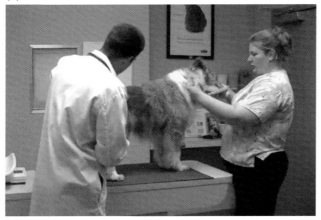

(c)

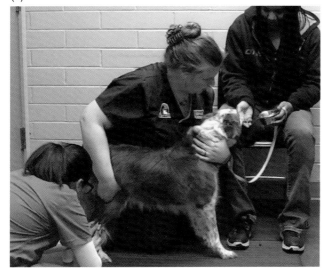

Figure 5.9 (a–c) Several options for lateral saphenous venipuncture using food distractions.

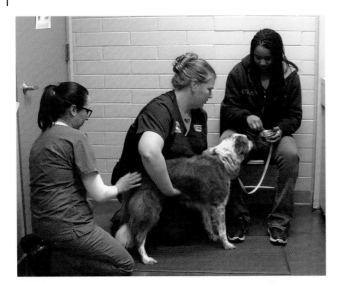

Figure 5.10 Begin touch near the hip, then glide to the venipuncture or injection area.

For both dogs and cats, assure the patient is sitting on a comfortable nonslip surface. One person will be helping the patient sit stationary and offering food, while a second person collects the sample. Assure the patient is accepting food or tactile rewards, and gently position the chin using both the location of the treats and a hand under the chin for stability. We do not recommend stretching patients over the end of the table. Once the patient is comfortable, occlude the vessel, palpate, apply alcohol, pinch the area lightly, then collect the sample. The technician who is stabilizing the patient should communicate any changes in food acceptance and body language. If the dog or cat struggles, let her move away and evaluate the handling plan.

Video 5.16 shows a black Labrador retriever, Skittles, participating in a jugular blood draw while eating baby food from a syringe. Monique invites Skittles onto the mat by luring her with the treats, then gently stabilizes under her chin. Skittles eats the baby food before, during, and after her blood draw.

Video 5.17 shows a low-restraint jugular blood draw on Kanga. She is an older Chihuahua, and we use minimal stabilization for her head. We provide food rewards immediately after the blood draw. We started by using food distractions during this procedure, but it caused her to move around too much, so we changed the timing to food following the blood draw. This is a good example of choosing the right strategy for each individual patient.

Blood Pressure Measurement

For blood pressure measurement using a Doppler or self-contained non-invasive blood pressure unit (NIBP), it is important to reduce stress as much as possible to obtain an accurate reading. Restraining the pet and causing anxiety or struggling will increase the patient's blood pressure reading, and can lead to false high readings.

Allow the patient to assume a comfortable position. This may be standing, sitting down, or lying down depending upon the pet. When possible, have the owner nearby to help the patient relax and cooperate, and even offer the treats. Once the patient is in a comfortable position, allow the patient to keep his limbs in the preferred position and apply the blood pressure cuff. Assess the patient for changes in food acceptance and body language. If the patient appears comfortable, hold the Doppler crystal to the artery. Use headphones to listen for the signal so the sound does not upset the patient. Once the signal is acquired, continue offering food and tactile rewards through the measurement and while the crystal and blood pressure cuff are removed.

Video 5.18 shows a Level One cat having her blood pressure measured while sitting in an owner's lap. This cat is not interested in food, but enjoys stroking and the owner speaking softly to her. The technician tries to disturb the cat's preferred position as little as possible during the measurement, and the cat remains relaxed through the procedure.

Cystocentesis

Cystocentesis is the gold standard for urine sample collection, but it may not be right for every patient. Positioning for cystocentesis can be stressful for patients, so choosing a plan appropriate to the patient is important. For patients who are stressed by cystocentesis, consider a sterile free-catch sample as a reasonable alternative.[2] If a free-catch culture is positive and there is a question of contamination, confirmatory cystocentesis can be scheduled if medically necessary, using appropriate anxiolytic or sedative medications.

Level One cats will often allow cystocentesis standing or in sternal recumbency rolled onto a hip in the same position used for medial saphenous venipuncture (Figure 5.11). The cat must have an easily palpated bladder for this procedure to be safe and simple. If the bladder is small or difficult to palpate, select another position for cystocentesis, or collect the sample at a better time when the bladder is more full. One technician should stabilize the cat, offering food and tactile distractions depending upon the cat's preference. The technician performing the cystocentesis will begin touching in a less sensitive area, such as over the back, then move to abdominal palpation. Isolate the bladder and move it laterally toward the flank, smoothing the skin over the bladder with your thumb. Assure no other intra-abdominal structures are between the bladder and the body wall. Once the bladder is well isolated, apply a small amount of alcohol, and perform the cystocentesis. Level One cats generally stand or sit nice and still throughout this procedure.

Cystocentesis for dogs requires slightly different positioning because the bladder is not as freely palpated and moved compared with cats. We encourage the use of ultrasound for canine cystocentesis.

For large Level One dogs with a full bladder, standing ultrasound-guided cystocentesis can be a low-stress procedure (Figure 5.12). One technician will stabilize the dog standing on a nonslip surface and offer treats, monitoring the dog's body language and food acceptance. A second technician can approach from beside the dog, sitting or kneeling on the floor. Begin by stroking the dog on his side or back, then touching the abdomen with a hand and then the ultrasound probe. Verify the bladder is full, and there are no other intra-abdominal structures between the bladder and the body wall.

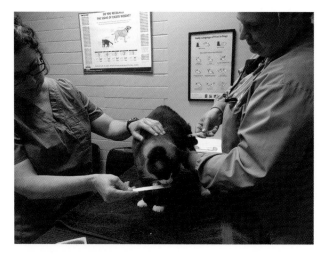

Figure 5.11 Positioning for Level One feline cystocentesis.

(a)

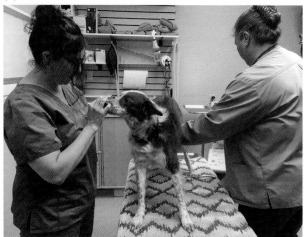

(b)

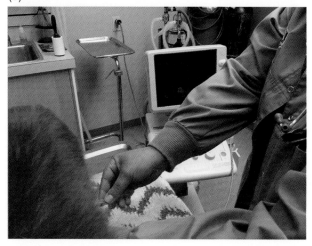

Figure 5.12 Positioning for Level One canine standing cystocentesis.

Introduce the needle and perform cystocentesis. Small and medium dogs may be gently placed in lateral or dorsal recumbency. Using similar strategies to those seen in the radiograph positioning videos, gently establish recumbency while offering pleasant food and tactile distractions. Using ultrasound, verify the bladder is full and appropriately positioned, then perform cystocentesis. If the dog is struggling or fearful about positioning or scanning, stop and allow the dog to move away, then make a new handling plan. Medical treatment of anxiety and stress is generally the most expedient means for obtaining cystocentesis for fearful animals. This is rarely a frequent or serial procedure, so investing the time and effort training specifically for cystocentesis may have diminishing returns.

5.6 Administering Medications and Grooming

Medication Stations

Often, we perform treatments in the hospital such as eye medication, ear medication, or oral medication, and then prescribe these same treatments to be continued in the home. Training a medication station will simplify treating pets at home. It is crucial, whenever we prescribe a treatment, that the method for how to complete the treatment is part of the prescription. The medication station is introduced in Chapter 4. The patient should be taught to target the desired location, be it a mat, a cushion, a bed, or another area. The station should be easy for the pet to recognize, and a location of much fun and reinforcement. Once the medication station has been taught, we can sometimes take "training shortcuts," relying on the positive power of the station to avoid having to desensitize every type of medication.

Video 5.19 shows Alicea asking Piper to go to the medication station. Piper is quite happy to do so, and accepts eye drops without any further training simply because the station is so enjoyable and has been conditioned in advance. If owners have taken the time to train a medication station, consider asking them to bring the mat or bed along to veterinary visits.

Video 5.20 demonstrates the same training process with a feline patient.

Oral Medications

Imagine you're sitting on a blanket at a lovely summer picnic, with a bowl of beautiful berries in your lap. As you eat the delicious berries, you encounter a lip-puckering eye-squinting sour berry. Ick! But the rest of the bowl beckons, and you try another berry even though one was sour. This is how we would like pets to think of oral medications. If they notice the "sour berry" at all, it happens infrequently enough compared to the delicious ones they will try again. However, if every time we give a special treat, there is a sour pill in the center, the patient may learn that the special food predicts the bitter pill, and will become wary of special treats.

Teach owners to disguise a pill in a food treat. Do not give pills in an entire meal, as this is just an invitation to eat around the pill and skip taking the medication. Clever pets will quickly make this decision. When preparing the pill, prepare 3–5 treats rather than just one. Select a treat the patient enjoys such as canned food, small meat pieces, cheese, cream cheese, or even commercially available pill-hiding treats. Offer one or two plain treats, then the medicated treat, and immediately offer one or two plain treats. Rapidly offering the plain treats will encourage the animal to eat the medicated treat rapidly to make room for the next food being offered. Video 5.21 demonstrates the multiple-treat method for giving a pill to a dog. Notice the technician gives the treats rapidly, encouraging the dog to swallow right away and not spend a lot of time thinking about what might or might not be hidden in them.

Liquid medications can often be mixed with delicious soft food. Starting young animals out accepting food from a syringe will prepare them to accept liquid medications in the future. If it is a small volume of medicine, it can often be mixed with a small amount of food and administered simply as a treat. If the volume of medicine is a bit larger, use an alternating syringe method, just as the 3–5 treat method is explained above. Load one syringe with delicious food, and one syringe with the medication mixed with a bit of delicious food. Begin by offering the syringe with the delicious food. Once the animal is licking the syringe well, change syringes and administer the medication, then change back right away to the plain delicious treat syringe. Going back to our analogy, the delicious sweet berries should outnumber the sour ones in any bowl.

This may sound like a lot of work! Consider how much time will be saved when patients willingly show up for medication rather than the owner having to chase pets all over their homes. Filling and washing two syringes is much more efficient than getting the medication ready, hunting down Fluffy who has run off and is hiding under the bed, dragging Fluffy out from under the bed, wrapping her in a blanket, prying her mouth open, spraying the medicine in, and then cleaning up the towel, the medication mess, putting the bed back where it belongs, and washing out the syringe.

Puppies and kittens can be taught from an early age to accept treats manually like a pill, and to eat treats from a syringe. Often when we give liquid treats in the clinic, we will administer them using a syringe because of the helpful effect it has of teaching animals how to enjoy accepting liquids from syringes.

Video 5.22 shows a puppy's first introduction to accepting treats in the same fashion as a pill, and accepting liquid food from a syringe simulating oral medications. Notice the puppy stays near the technician, has relaxed body language, and continues accepting food throughout the training session.

Video 5.23 shows a young kitten learning to accept liquid medications from a syringe. Notice Alicea switches between the syringe holding only delicious food and the syringe with the mixture of medicine and food to keep the kitten engaged and willing to participate.

Ear Medications and Cleaning

Level One dogs and cats will often allow ear cleaning and placement of medication using a distraction method without restraint. *If the animal has a painful infected ear, please move to Level Two training.* Using distraction methods for animals with painful conditions will often poison the distraction. The food begins to predict something painful occurring, so the animal learns not to take food in that circumstance, rather than learning to tolerate and enjoy handling and treatment.

Use a distraction such as sticky treats on a spoon, a toy or bowl with canned food, or treats smeared on a vertical surface. Help the animal stand, sit, or lie down comfortably. Once the animal is eating, touch a less sensitive area such as the shoulder. Glide up to the base of the ear, then lift the ear flap. Using a wet cotton ball or cleansing pad, apply cleanser and then massage the ear canal. The animal will generally stop eating during this moment, and then shake his head. If the animal returns to eating right away, continue with the ear cleansing. If the animal's body language, food acceptance, and proximity preference indicate increasing stress levels, change to Level Two training described in Chapter 6.

Video 5.24 shows Alicea using a spoon with sticky food as a distraction while she places ear medication for greyhound Honu. The distraction is very effective, and he tolerates the procedure well.

Nail Trims

Nail trimming is a fact of life in the veterinary hospital, but why? We are not groomers, and this is a basic part of animal husbandry just like feeding or brushing. Nail trims are almost never a medical emergency, but they can permanently damage the relationship between the veterinary team and the pet. Animals have sensitive paws, and often they have had negative experiences where a huge wrestling match predicts a nail trim, and perhaps even pain when a nail is trimmed too short. Remember, even dogs and cats who have never had a painful nail trim can find nail trims stressful, so prevention and Level One training are important to get this grooming procedure started out on the right paw. Level One training is only appropriate if the patient has no previous unpleasant learning history and negative emotional response. To reverse an existing problem, please refer to Level Two and Level Three. No dog ever "needs" to be put into lateral recumbency for grooming. No cat "needs" to be scruffed and stretched for a nail trim. These animals deserve medical and behavioral treatment of fear and anxiety prior to grooming, rather than to be subjected to a non-emergency, nonmedical procedure that can damage the trust between veterinary team and patient forever.

Training Tip: Remember the 2-2-3 Rule!
Two gentle stabilizing arms Two seconds of struggling for cats Three seconds of struggling for dogs Any more than this requires a pause, assessment, and new training plan.

For Level One patients, allow the dog or cat to choose a comfortable position. Standing is generally the easiest position to access all the paws and provide food distractions. Very small dogs sometimes prefer to be held in someone's arms or sit on the owner's lap during nail trims. Some cats prefer to sit in a carrier bottom. One technician (or the owner, depending upon your hospital policy) should provide food distractions while a technician works to provide the grooming. Begin touching in a less sensitive area such as the shoulder, then glide down to the elbow, carpus, paw, toe, toenail, and then clip. Raise the paw into a natural walking or reaching position, avoid lifting the leg too high or off to the side (Figure 5.13). If the patient struggles, has an increase in anxious body language, or stops accepting food, pause the procedure. If pausing the procedure does not result in an immediate return to baseline, consider changing to Level Two or Level Three training.

(a)

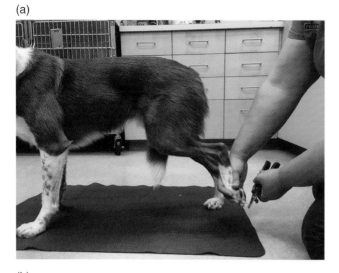

(b)

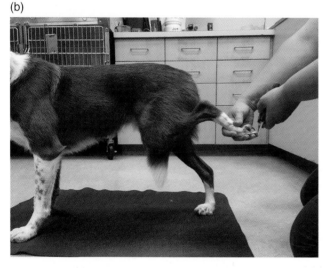

Figure 5.13 (a) Correct paw positioning for a standing canine nail trim. The paw should be held low in a comfortable walking position. (b) Incorrect paw position.

Preventive desensitization and classical conditioning can also be used for Level One dogs and cats, especially puppies and kittens. Desensitization and classical conditioning have an advantage over distraction techniques because the food distraction is unlikely to begin predicting the nail trim, so the patient won't become wary of food offered in the hospital. The primary difference between the distraction method and the classical conditioning method is timing. For the distraction method, the food is offered before, during, and after the procedure. With desensitization and classical conditioning, touch *predicts* the food, so it is provided after each step in the process, but not during the handling.

 Video 5.25 shows the distraction technique for an elderly Dachshund. This dog was presented with extremely overgrown toenails because the owner stated nail trims were

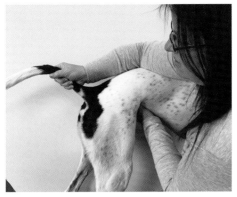

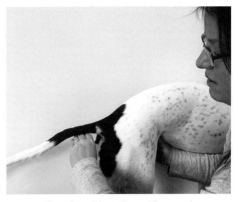

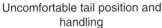

Uncomfortable tail position and handling

Comfortable tail position and handling

Figure 5.14 Correct and incorrect tail position for temperature measurement or anal gland expression.

a huge battle, and very stressful. With some patience and good planning, this dog received a low-stress nail trim while eating peanut butter from a spoon. Notice the dog is comfortable eating before, during, and after the nail trim, and the veterinary team is providing support but not restraint.

Video 5.26 demonstrates preventive desensitization and classical conditioning. The goal of nail trimming is broken down into numerous small steps as discussed in Chapter 3. Each small step predicts a click and treat. The puppy begins offering his paws and impatiently trying to participate in the nail trim while the owner watches, learning how to replicate the technique at home with her puppy.

Anal Gland Expression

Anal gland expression is rarely medically necessary, but often a grooming request from the owner. This means it is almost always a want, and almost never a need. Using lidocaine jelly as lubricant can assist in making anal gland expression more comfortable, but this procedure understandably provokes strong responses in many patients. As with temperature measurement, assure the tail is lifted mildly, and not excessively, to reduce patient discomfort (Figure 5.14). Because of the strong response many patients have, Level One training is almost never appropriate for anal gland expression. Refer to Level Two and Level Three for strategies to condition pets to accept this procedure.

Conclusion

Level One training should be the basic standard of care for most patients who do not have a preexisting fear response, do not have a painful condition, and will not require repeated treatments. The proper application of distractions and gentle support allows many relaxed patients to receive care with little or even no physical restraint for both traditional and complementary therapies (see feline acupuncture using this method in

Video 5.27). If the patient is anxious, stressed, or fearful; has a painful condition such as otitis or arthritis; or will require the treatment repeatedly, such as insulin injections; Level Two and Level Three training are more appropriate choices.

References

1 Reichart, P. (1984) Periodontal disease in the domestic cat: A histopathological study. *Journal of Periodontal Research.* 19 (1), 67–75.
2 Weese, J. (2011) Antimicrobial use guidelines for treatment of urinary tract disease in dogs and cats: Antimicrobial Guidelines Working Group of the International Society for Companion Animal Infectious Diseases. *Veterinary Medicine International.* 2011 (2011), art. ID 263768. https://doi.org/10.4061/2011/263768

6

Level Two Patients and Training

6.1 Level Two Training

Training for Level Two patients goes beyond using distraction techniques. Level Two training is appropriate for Level Two and Level One patients, but not for Level Three patients. Remember: setting up the environment for success is still crucial. Check the medical record for individual preferences, set up the working area in a relaxing way from the pet's point of view, and remember to consistently assess and reassess the patient throughout the visit, pausing to make a new plan if necessary.

Referring to Chapters 3 and 4, you will recall the procedures of desensitization, classical conditioning, and classical counterconditioning. Level Two patients will benefit from these techniques. Some Level Two patients are naturally shy or wary of new experiences, may be naturally fearful of restraint, or have had a learning history of fear-provoking veterinary procedures in the past. Rather than prevention, as is the case with most Level One patients, Level Two patients need intervention to reverse their fear and anxiety, and prevent it from worsening over time. When making a training plan for a Level Two patient, we will need to identify the assessment protocol for Level Two patients and determine if desensitization and classical conditioning or counterconditioning are the tools of choice. We can then make a desensitization hierarchy and classical conditioning or counterconditioning plan to improve the patient's ability to tolerate the procedure, remain in a positive emotional state, and cooperate during medical treatment.

Some Level Two patients will need to have training visits prior to the completion of a service, such as a physical examination. The methods described in this chapter can be used during a primary visit, during training preparation visits, or both. Veterinary technicians with the right skills are extremely valuable, because we can provide training visits to prepare patients for better care from the veterinarian. Many of the videos in this chapter are from training visits used to ready the patient for more in-depth veterinary care.

6.2 Identifying Level Two Patients

Patient assessment requires us to be flexible as observers. Patients may switch between levels at any time in the process, and there is fluidity in their behaviors. The structure of these assessments is a basic guideline. In general, Level Two patients are experiencing mild or moderate stress as described in Chapter 2. These patients often find the

Cooperative Veterinary Care, First Edition. Alicea Howell and Monique Feyrecilde.
© 2018 John Wiley & Sons, Inc. Published 2018 by John Wiley & Sons, Inc.
Companion website: www.wiley.com/go/howell/cooperative

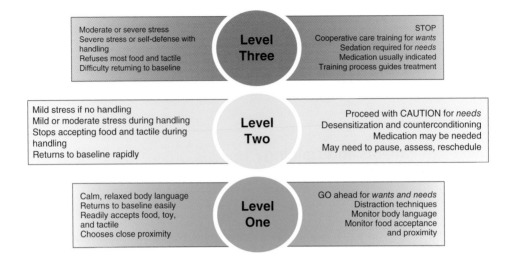

Figure 6.1 Evaluation guide for Level Two patients.

environment or the procedure mildly fear provoking, but not severely. When patients are experiencing moderate stress levels, it is difficult for them to learn new skills or form positive emotional responses. If the fight-or-flight response gets triggered, the patient will move into self-defense or self-preservation mode, and the good window for learning will close. Part of Level Two training will be to interact with the patient in a way that improves their emotional status and decreases anxiety and fear, so they can learn the veterinary skills more effectively (Figure 6.1).

Many Level Two patients will benefit from medical management of fear and stress. From neutraceuticals and pheromones to anxiety-reducing pharmaceuticals, many options are available for the medical treatment of veterinary anxiety. For truly stress-free care, consider using event-based treatments prior to veterinary visits. Over time, if the owner pursues training, the dosage can often be decreased or the medication weaned entirely away; but the patient experience should be a top priority for the veterinary team, and for some patients, "Medicine is the best medicine."

Training Tip: Drugs Not Hugs!

Medicine is often the best medicine, not more restraint. Be sure to provide medical intervention for fear, stress, and anxiety whenever indicated. Early intervention treating fear is always more effective than attempts to reverse severe anxiety once it has already begun.

Level Two Dogs

Food Acceptance
- Dogs will accept food immediately or after <5 seconds
- Will accept high-value food from any team member
- Will accept lower value food from trusted or preferred team members
- Takes food with a soft mouth; no snapping or grabbing when no handling is occurring
- May begin taking food roughly when handling or procedures begin

- May continue taking food or may stop taking food during procedures
- If stopped accepting food during the procedure, may accept a higher value food
- If stopped taking food during handling or procedure, immediately begins taking food again when the handling or procedure is completed

Table 6.1 provides a quick reference checklist for assessing Level Two dogs. Figure 6.2 shows a Level Two dog.

Table 6.1 Checklist for Level Two dogs: Each dog assessing at Level Two may have a combination of these attributes.

Stage of visit	Food acceptance	Body language	Proximity preference
Greeting	☐ High-value from any team member ☐ Low-value from preferred people or owner ☐ Within 5 seconds ☐ Soft mouth	☐ Relaxed body	☐ Greets immediately ☐ Stays near team member ☐ May or may not solicit attention
Touching	☐ High-value treats only ☐ May take treat roughly	☐ Mild tension during touch	☐ Moves away ☐ Moves toward owner
Exam & treatment	☐ High-value treats only ☐ May take treat roughly	☐ Mild tension during procedures ☐ Returns to baseline <10 seconds	☐ Does not move away ☐ Remains close during treatments ☐ Returns to baseline <10 seconds

Figure 6.2 Level Two canine patient.

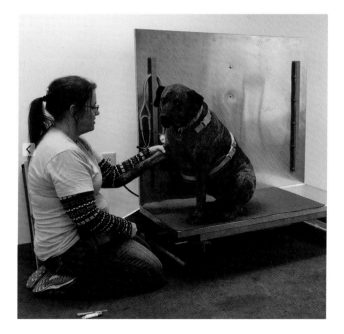

Body Language
- Relaxed body language in the hospital when not being handled (refer to Chapter 2)
- May show mild stress markers during handling:
  - Looking or leaning away
  - Mild pupil dilation
  - Closed mouth or increased respiratory rate (refer to Chapter 2)
  - Moving away when procedure begins or is attempted
  - Attention seeking from the owner but not veterinary team members
  - Tense muscles or exaggerated panniculus response when touched
  - Tail is tense or held abnormally low for the breed
- May show mild to moderate stress markers during procedures
- When the handling and procedure are stopped, returns to baseline relaxed state within 10 seconds

Proximity Preference
- Off-leash, dog immediately greets veterinary team members
- Chooses to remain near team members while they talk to and touch him
- May retreat closer to the owner, back away, or move away when approached
- May choose to stay near team members when approached, but show other signs of stress simultaneously
- Will retreat closer to the owner, back away, or move away when touched
- Tries to move away during procedures
- Will return to baseline proximity preference within 10 seconds of stopping procedures

Level Two Cats

As mentioned in this book, food acceptance is a less reliable indicator of stress in cats when contrasted against dogs. However, for cats who will eat in the hospital, changes in food acceptance are a useful indicator of stress levels.

Food Acceptance, Toy Acceptance, and Tactile Acceptance
- Investigates or accepts food while in carrier, or within 30 seconds of exiting carrier
- Interacts with toy if toy motivated
- Investigates offered food, but may or may not eat depending upon preferences
- Accepts food before touching, but ceases eating or eats more roughly during touching
- Stops eating during procedures
- May return to eating after procedures, or show interest in food and then choose not to eat
- May show interest in tactile rewards such as chin and cheek rubs
- May stop tactile acceptance during procedures, but rapidly returns to baseline after procedure

Body Language
- Relaxed body language after exiting carrier and before handling (refer to Chapter 2)
- Mild stress markers during handling, such as:
  - Moving slowly and cautiously
  - Whiskers pulled forward
  - Ears to the side

■ Increased respiratory rate (refer to Chapter 2)
■ Purring without soliciting attention
■ Slightly tense muscles when touched; exaggerated panniculus response
■ Tail tucked close to body
■ Paws concealed when lying down
- Mild stress markers during procedures
- Returns to baseline body language within 30 seconds of completion of procedure

Proximity Preference
- Chooses to exit carrier within 1 minute of arrival
- May explore exam room but cautiously, crouching or following walls
- May choose to sit stationary near the owner or in a neutral location
- May approach team members, but may not
- Does not retreat when team members approach without attempting handling
- Allows facial petting and stroking before handling or procedures
- Attempts to move away when handling begins
- Attempts to move away during procedures
- Returns to baseline proximity preference within 30 seconds of completing procedures

Table 6.2 provides a quick reference checklist for assessing Level Two cats. Figure 6.3 shows a Level Two cat.

Patients who are appropriate for Level Two training are either relaxed or mildly stressed in the veterinary environment. Their stress level generally increases slightly during handling and procedures, but they are capable of returning to baseline after handling and procedures. Level Two training is a combination of helping the animal to relax, and then teaching the patient that the veterinary procedure is nonthreatening and is associated with pleasurable things.

Remember: health status and individual preference influence assessment and training levels. Any patient known to have a painful condition such as an ear infection, lameness, or gastrointestinal (GI) upset should be assumed to need Level Two protocols at minimum. Using a little bit of extra proactive planning for these patients will increase success

Table 6.2 Checklist for Level Two cats: Each cat assessing at Level Two may have a combination of these attributes.

Stage of visit	Food or tactile acceptance	Body language	Proximity preference
Greeting	☐ Shows some interest ☐ May eat within 30 seconds ☐ May prefer toy ☐ May prefer tactile	☐ Relaxed body	☐ Exits carrier willingly ☐ Explores exam room ☐ Solicits attention
Touching	☐ Desire diminished by touch ☐ Return to baseline <30 seconds	☐ Moderate stress markers	☐ Moves away ☐ Return to baseline <30 seconds
Exam & treatment	☐ Desire diminished by touch ☐ Return to baseline <30 seconds	☐ Moderate stress markers	☐ Moves away ☐ Return to baseline <30 seconds

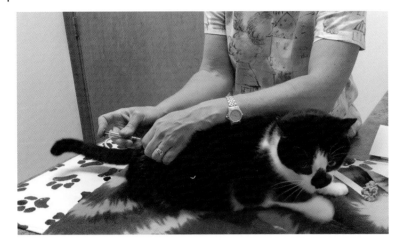

Figure 6.3 Level Two feline patient.

and decrease unwanted outcomes over time. Often, Level Two patients can have their exam and procedures done during a single visit. In some cases, these patients need to be rescheduled to allow either medical management of stress and anxiety, or training prior to proceeding with nonvital treatments. When attempting Level Two training with patients, notify the veterinarian right away if the patient's fear and stress seem to be worsening rather than improving, so the patient can be reassessed and a new plan formulated.

6.3   Level Two Training: Dog Exam Room and Examination

Level Two dogs may show mild to moderate stress in the reception area and on the way to the exam room. Signs can change rapidly, so be watchful, and continue to do things like offering treats repeatedly even if the dog refuses them. Often dogs who initially refuse food will decide to accept it as time passes. Also, offering different treats and using different approaches can enhance food acceptance. Level Two dogs may not feel comfortable taking treats from your hand or a spoon, but may follow a treat trail or accept treats from the owner's hand. As these dogs are slightly more stressed, they are more susceptible to trigger stacking. The more stressed an animal is, the less emotional energy they have available to tolerate time and events within the hospital. We need to plan to provide services in order of importance to make the best use of the patient's ability to cooperate.

Reception, Weight, and Moving to the Exam Room

The customer service team member or veterinary technician should calmly greet the dog, allowing the dog to approach if he chooses to. If the dog chooses not to approach, dropping a few treats onto the floor and turning away may help the dog feel more confident. If the dog will follow a treat trail onto the scale, collect a body weight. If the dog is too nervous to be weighed easily, consider postponing the weight until after the examination at the end of the visit.

To invite the dog into the exam room, try using a treat trail or a lure as described for Level One patients in Chapter 5. If the dog is too nervous to accept food, stops moving, or begins backing up, stop trying to move the dog and instruct the owner how to make a treat trail or how to hold the lure. Move out of the way, preferably to a point behind the dog so the entrance to the exam room is clear, and see if the owner can invite the dog into the exam room. Coach the owner to keep the leash loose, and observe the dog's ability to follow the lure. If the dog is reluctant to follow, try having the owner offer higher value treats, give treats more frequently or place treats closer together, or toss the treats so they are exciting to chase. Figure 6.4 shows an example of using treat placement on the floor of the exam room to promote patient movement.

If this plan fails, do not drag the dog into the examination room. This dog may be best examined in the lobby, the parking lot, or the car for today, and signed up for happy visits or Level Three training for moving into the exam room in the future. Stressing the dog excessively over trying to enter the exam room may sabotage your ability to provide an exam or other treatments by using up the dog's emotional reserves before they ever step into the room.

Some dogs who are moderately fearful approaching the scale or examination room may be nervous about the texture or sheen of the floors. Rolling out a few rugs or yoga mats to make a good-traction trail into the exam room sometimes makes all the difference for dogs who are sensitive to slick or shiny floors. If you're not sure, ask the owner. Many owners are aware their dogs fear slippery floors, but it doesn't occur to them that this is the reason the dog is reluctant to move through the lobby or exam room.

Video 6.1 shows a dog who is too nervous to enter the exam room. Alicea shows the owner how easy it is to use food lures to move the nervous dog forward. Notice that Alicea uses a jackpot of several treats once the dog is in the exam room as a reward.

The Exam Room

Mildly stressed dogs will still usually approach the technician. Greeting these dogs in a nonthreatening way is crucial. Sit in a chair next to the owner, or on the floor with your side to the dog. Begin by tossing treats away from you to encourage the dog to move around the room. Each time he approaches you, mark with a click or a verbal marker, then toss the treat away. By feeding away from where we are sitting, we are resetting the dog to practice approaches several times and giving him a chance to relax in between approaches. Usually these dogs will approach closer and closer, and after only a few repetitions will try to take food from a hand held low, below their nose level. Once the dog is taking treats from a hand held low, gently reach and offer to touch the dog on his chest between his front legs, as with the Level One greeting. Once you've initiated touch, immediately treat. Repeat the touch–treat, touch–treat, touch–treat process several times. If using a clicker, the order is touch, click while touching, stop touching, treat. The goal is to establish that *touch **predicts** food*, rather than using food as a distraction or to convince the dog to stick around for touching. Level Two dogs are often suspicious if food is offered and then we try to reach out with a second hand to touch. Use the principles of classical conditioning rather than distractions for these Level Two patients. Table 6.3 shows a worksheet for planning and tracking the desensitization and counterconditioning (DS/CC) process.

While questioning the owner regarding the medical history for the day's visit, and greeting the Level Two dog, the technician should begin to assess where the dog will be

(a)

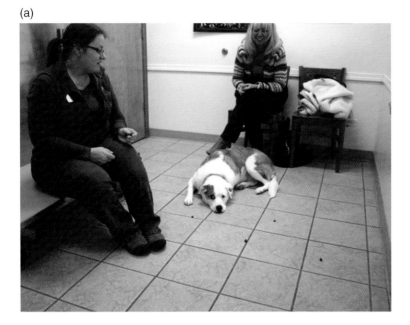

(b)

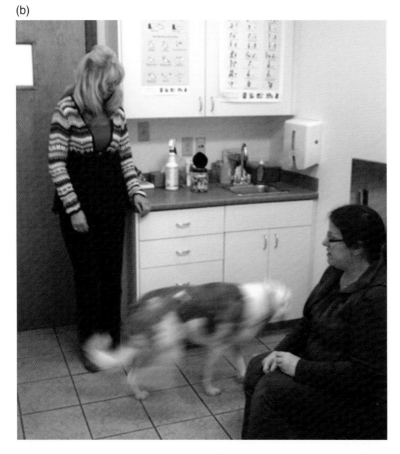

Figure 6.4 (a) A treat trail on the floor and (b) having the owner move can encourage fearful dogs to explore.

Table 6.3 Desensitization and counterconditioning worksheet: A basic template for setting up a DS/CC/CCC plan for a patient.

Training plan: Desensitization and counterconditioning	
Trigger:	Exposure ladder:
Foundation behaviors required:	
Preferred rewards to generate positive emotional response 1. 2. 3.	
Medications:	Working area:
Nonstressful starting point:	
Distance	
Duration	
Pressure	
Volume	
Other	
Endpoint	
Homework	
Plan for next visit	

Source: Available for download in the Online Resources.

most comfortable for the examination. Most large Level Two dogs will respond negatively to team members trying to lift them onto the table and should be examined on the floor. Many small Level Two dogs will allow lifting to the table with a rapid desensitization protocol.

Table Training

To desensitize and countercondition the table, we need to make a desensitization hierarchy, or exposure ladder. For a small dog, the completed behavior will be "Allow a technician to pick you up and place you on the table." To make the exposure ladder, we need to break down the pick-up behavior into its component parts. For counterconditioning, we need to make sure every baby step up the ladder predicts something wonderful from the dog's point of view: something that evokes a pleasant emotional response (Figure 6.5).

Example exposure ladder for placing a small dog on the table:

- Dog approaches handler, indicating a nonstressful starting point.
- Dog allows handler to touch between the front legs.
- Dog allows handler to squat beside while touching between the front legs.
- Dog allows handler to squat, touch, and reach slightly over the back.
- Dog allows handler to reach over the back and touch the opposite side.
- Dog allows handler to reach over, touch, and then reach under the chest.
- Dog allows handler to reach over, reach under, and squeeze dog against her thigh.

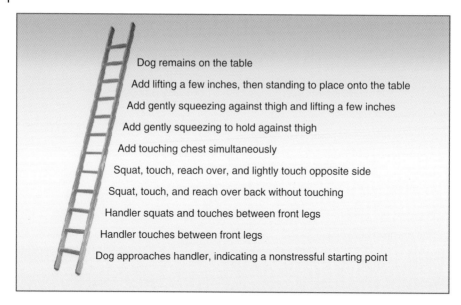

Figure 6.5 Example exposure ladder for table training.

- Dog allows handler to squeeze against her thigh and lift a few inches.
- Dog allows handler to lift a few inches, then stand up and place on the table.
- Dog remains on the table.

Every one of these baby steps should *predict* a *wonderful* treat the dog wants and willingly accepts. Remember: if the patient's stress level increases, pause the process and let the animal rest for a moment, then try again from the most recent nonstressful rung on the ladder.

Training Tip: Exposure Ladders are Always Under Construction!

Remember: exposure ladders are not set in stone. They are flexible and can be deconstructed, modified, or reconfigured at any time.

You might go up the ladder and down the ladder in a few repetitions, you may have to add rungs if an approximation causes stress, or you may be able to skip rungs if the patient is comfortable and relaxed.

Video 6.2 demonstrates how to rapidly desensitize and countercondition a small dog to allow lifting onto the table. This process took about 30 seconds, and the dog had a pleasant experience. Notice the technician makes sure the dog will approach; breaks down the process of lifting into a series of baby steps, with each step predicting a tasty treat; then makes sure the dog will remain on the table for treats.

This dog has been presented for a nail trim. After the table training and pick-up training, the puppy is still showing signs of moderate stress. The technician takes the time to educate the owner about what she is seeing, and the owner asks if it would be better to do the nail trim another day after some training. What a terrific interaction!

Physical Examination

For the Level Two dog, the less time spent handling, the less stress the dog will experience. Communication is vital. Either during the history, or when the veterinarian comes into the room to greet the client and patient, time should be taken to educate the client about the patient's stress level, and how this will guide the handling plan for the day. Consider the following script: "Mrs. Smith, I see Fluffy is a bit nervous to be here today. We will do our best to help her feel comfortable by teaching her the exam is nothing to fear. If she becomes too nervous, we will stop what we are doing, but we are going to try and complete her exam as quickly as possible. Once we are done with her exam, we can discuss our findings while Fluffy has a chance to relax."

The order of the physical examination should be much as it is in Chapter 5, with the least invasive touches performed first, always starting in a less sensitive area first and moving to more sensitive areas. The oral exam, paw handling, rectal exam, and any painful areas should be examined last. The position of the veterinarian to the side of the patient most of the time should also remain the same, avoiding face-to-face potentially confrontational body language unless the dog clearly prefers this approach. The main difference between a Level One and a Level Two examination is the change from distraction training to desensitization and counterconditioning.

For a Level Two exam, the process will need to be broken down into baby steps, just like table training. Each baby step should predict a wonderful treat. Recall that for desensitization, we control the intensity of the trigger. Controlling intensity of the exam portions can include softening touches getting gradually more firm, small touches such as with a finger covering a larger surface area with more fingers or a whole hand, brief touches becoming lengthier, or gliding a touch from a less sensitive to more sensitive area.

The role of the veterinary technician is to monitor the patient's response, provide well-timed treats in coordination with the veterinarian's examination to facilitate desensitization and counterconditioning, and alert the veterinarian to changes in the dog's stress level during examination. It is important that each step on the exposure ladder predicts something wonderful. Also, each exposure ladder example we provide is simply an example. The steps may need to be changed in order, or modified in difficulty or duration depending upon the needs of the individual patient. With practice and good patient observation, modifying exposure ladders can become second nature.

Example exposure ladder for a Level Two physical exam:

- Allow the dog to find a comfortable position as the nonstressful starting point
- Touch shoulder
- Touch shoulder, glide along spine
- Glide along spine, down **flank**
- Glide down flank, examine ventrum for 2 seconds
- Extend to 5 seconds
- Present stethoscope
- Place hand on auscultation location
- Approach touch point with stethoscope
- Auscult for 2 seconds, then for 5 seconds
- Auscult for gradually longer periods until completed
- Glide one hand to the abdomen
- Add a second hand to the abdomen

- Palpate gently
- Palpate deeply for 2 seconds
- Palpate deeply for progressively longer intervals
- Palpate lymph nodes
  - May need to make subsets of 1–2 lymph nodes at a time
- Palpate limbs one at a time, each one counting as a step on the ladder
  - The limbs may need to be subsets of a joint at a time
- Examine the external ear
  - Divide the ear exam into **pinna**, visual outer canal, opening canal with a finger
- Examine each eye
  - If necessary, reach toward the upper eyelid on one side
  - Touch the upper eyelid
  - Repeat steps for the second side
- Oral exam
  - Touch the nose
  - Touch the lateral aspect of the upper lip
  - Raise the lip to expose the canine tooth
  - Raise the lip to expose the canine tooth, then stretch the lip backward to expose caudal teeth
  - Repeat for the second side
  - Gently add a second hand to the muzzle
  - Carefully open the mouth if patient is relaxed enough
- Examine limbs by touching the shoulder or hip first, then:
  - Elbow/**Stifle**
    - **Carpus/Hock**
    - Paw
    - Toe, Toenail
- Rectal and genital visual exam

Remember: every approximation should *predict* a wonderful treat. If the patient's stress level is increasing through the examination, consider postponing part of the examination to provide medical management of anxiety and training visits before trying again. Veterinary technicians with the right skills can desensitize the dog to portions of the (or the entire) physical examination over a series of visits, then the examination skills can be transferred to the doctor.

6.4   Level Two Training: Cat Exam Room and Examination

Level Two cats are mildly stressed, but still accepting food or toys, and tactile rewards such as facial grooming. Often, Level Two cats will benefit from medical treatment of anxiety prior to visits.

If a cat has a conditioned response to the cat carrier, desensitization and counterconditioning are indicated. Using a combination of desensitization and operant conditioning, cats can learn to enter their carriers and enjoy the cat carrier (Figure 6.6). Sometimes, an aspect of habituation (the intensity of the stimulus stays the same rather than being modified) is also required at the beginning of the training process.

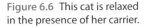

Figure 6.6 This cat is relaxed in the presence of her carrier.

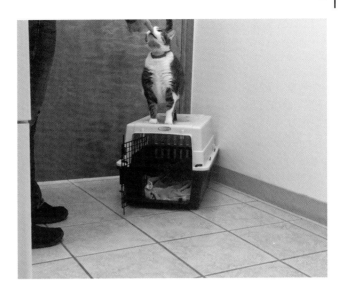

Training a cat to like and enter the carrier involves determining something the cat likes, such as canned food, cream cheese, butter, tuna flakes, or semi-moist cat treats. As with dogs, cats can learn the clicker predicts a wonderful food treat. We can then use the clicker to mark desired behavior, following up with the treat. Here are examples of multipurpose approximations for desensitization, classical counterconditioning, and shaping using operant conditioning to enter the carrier voluntarily.

Each approximation listed in this section, and any progress toward the carrier, earn a click and a treat. Give one treat near the carrier, then give a second treat 12 to 18 inches away from the carrier to reset the cat for a new opportunity to try the approach. Each step should be repeated a few times before criteria are increased. The length of this process depends upon the previous conditioned emotional response, how eager the cat is, the skill of the trainer, and the duration the cat chooses to remain engaged and working. The more intense the existing negative emotional response, the more patience and time will be required for desensitization. If there is a considerable negative response already, consider using a different carrier or dismantling the carrier and only using the bottom half to begin the training process. Try to stop training sessions before the cat chooses to opt out, instead ending on a positive note when the cat is still interested and happy.

Examples of approximations to desensitize, countercondition, and shape a carrier entrance:

- Establish a nonstressful starting point where the cat doesn't notice the carrier
- Remain in room where carrier is located
- Glance at carrier
  - Short glance, longer glance, look >3 seconds
- Glance at carrier, and then take one step toward it
  - Two steps, three steps, and so on until next to the carrier
- Sniff the carrier, or explore it by touching it
  - Sniff or touch the half with the door
  - Sniff or touch the end with the door
  - Sniff or touch the door opening

- Place nose in door opening
- Place head in door opening
- Place one paw inside carrier
  - Place two paws, then three paws, then four paws inside carrier
- Walk entirely inside the carrier and remain there for 2–3 seconds
- Walk into the carrier and remain there while the door is closed briefly
- Exit the carrier when the door is opened without increase in anxiety or flight.

Video 6.3 demonstrates using a combination of desensitization, classical conditioning, and shaping to teach a cat to voluntarily enter the carrier.

Cats who have been trained to enter the carrier will be happier and more relaxed when they arrive at the hospital. As with Level One, escort cats to the exam room promptly to avoid stressors in the reception area.

The Exam Room

As with the dog exam, Level Two cat exams are similar except that instead of distractions, they incorporate desensitization and classical counterconditioning. For success, the cat needs to be relaxed enough in the hospital to accept food, toys, or desired tactile rewards. If the cat is too fearful or anxious to accept food, toys, or tactile rewards, or will not approach team members nor allow handling without trying to move away or escape, consider providing medical management for anxiety before continuing. Every interaction with a patient is a learning experience, and we want them to learn not to fear us!

For Level Two cats who are accepting food, follow a similar procedure as for greeting dogs. For cats who are not accepting food, continue to offer it. Smelling the delicious food can serve as reinforcement, and food acceptance may improve over time. When the cat approaches, toss a small piece of food a few feet away (about two cat body lengths). With each subsequent approach, the cat will likely come closer and closer. When the cat chooses to greet, offer attention by stroking the cheek or along the spine, avoiding the top of the head or the sides and flanks. Reach out with one hand to pet, and then follow the touch with a treat. Each brief touch should *predict* a tiny delicious treat, to begin classically conditioning the cat to accept and enjoy touch in the exam room. If the cat prefers to sit with the owner, or remain in the bottom of the carrier, offer treats periodically and watch for signs of relaxation. Attempt a brief touch of the cheek or along the spine, and immediately provide a small delicious treat. If the cat chooses to remain stationary, continue. If the cat moves away or shows body language signs of increasing stress, stop touching at that time. If the cat is actively trying to hide, make sure to provide a hiding place such as a towel, a box, carrier lid placed back over the cat, or a bed with high sides.

While taking the history, assess where the cat seems most comfortable, and plan for the examination to be performed there. This may be on the exam table, on the floor, in the owner's lap, in a team member's lap, on a bench beside the owner, or the like. Comfortable cats are more cooperative.

Physical Examination

The physical examination can be broken down for desensitization and classical counterconditioning for cats in the same way as for dogs. Explain to the owner the importance of a rapid examination to decrease stress and increase the positive aspects of the patient's visit, and plan to discuss findings once the exam is completed and the patient is more comfortable. Each step of the physical examination should *predict* delicious food, a few seconds of toy play, or preferred tactile rewards such as cheek or chin stroking. Remember: most cats prefer to be approached from the side rather than face-to-face. A similar exposure ladder as what is suggested for dogs can be effective for cats as well.

Training Tip: Pause, Rewind, Playback in Slow Motion

During desensitization and classical conditioning or counterconditioning, the patient should look calm and relaxed. If you see a change in food acceptance, body language, or proximity preference, hit the pause button. Rewind the process to the most recent non-stressful point, and proceed in slow motion through the approximations, adding rungs to the exposure ladder if needed and assuring the patient remains comfortable and relaxed.

Example examination exposure ladder:

- Find a nonstressful starting position
- Stroke the cheek to establish touch
  - Stroke neck
  - Stroke chin; evaluate thyroid gland
  - Stroke shoulders
  - Follow midline along the spine
  - Stroke from the spine ventrally
- Evaluate lymph nodes while stroking the body
  - Each body region should be considered an approximation
- Touch the spine over the shoulders; glide laterally and ventrally to the sternum
- Touch the side of the chest where the stethoscope will touch the patient
- Place the stethoscope next to the hand touching the chest
  - Auscult for 3 seconds
  - Auscult progressively longer until complete
- Remove stethoscope, and glide hand to the abdomen
- Add a second hand to the abdomen if two hands are used to palpate
  - Alternatively, add a stabilizing hand elsewhere if single-hand palpation is used
- Palpate limbs one at a time, each one counting as a step on the ladder
  - The limbs may need to be subsets of a joint at a time
- Examine the external ear
  - Divide the ear exam into pinna, visual outer canal, opening canal with a finger
- Examine each eye
  - If necessary, reach toward the upper eyelid on one side
  - Touch the upper eyelid
  - Repeat steps for the second side
- Oral exam
  - Touch the nose
  - Touch the lateral aspect of the upper lip
  - Raise the lip to expose the canine tooth
  - Raise the lip to expose the canine tooth, then stretch the lip backward to expose caudal teeth
  - Glide finger to the lower lip to expose mandibular premolars and canine

- Repeat for the second side
- Gently add a second hand to the head
- Carefully open the mouth if patient is relaxed enough
- Examine limbs by touching the shoulder or hip first, then:
  - Elbow/Stifle
  - Carpus/Hock
  - Paw
  - Toe, Toenail
- Rectal and genital visual exam.

6.5 Level Two Training: Injections and Sample Collection

For Level Two patients, again dogs and cats are similar. With any patient, observe the pet closely for changes in food acceptance, body language, and proximity preference. If the pet's stress level is increasing during the visit, pause and assess the situation. Assure the treatment being performed is truly a want and not a need. If it is a need, notify the veterinarian that the patient is stressed, and obtain permission to give anxiety-relieving medications. If the procedure is a want, discuss a handling plan with the veterinarian for later in the day or another visit.

For procedures involving injections or needle sticks, the use of a topical cream anesthetic such as lidocaine–prilocaine can facilitate the procedure (also great for skin scrapings, ear treatments, rectal exams, and so much more!). With a gloved hand, massage the cream into the injection area and wait a few seconds before inserting the needle. If you wish to use topical cream, make sure to incorporate this step into your exposure ladder.

Subcutaneous and Intramuscular Injection

Level Two patients benefit from desensitization and counterconditioning for subcutaneous injections. The process may take as little as a few seconds, or as much as a few visits for the pet to be truly comfortable. Desensitization always progresses at the patient's rate. If we allow the animals to communicate with us, and we pay attention to what they are trying to say, we can gain trust and form positive emotional responses to injections as well as other procedures. Desensitization and classical conditioning or counterconditioning should not only be practiced in the hospital, but also be demonstrated to every pet owner when an injectable medication is prescribed such as insulin.

As with the exam, table training, carrier training, and more, desensitization for injections begins with finding a nonstressful starting point. Next, each step along the exposure ladder will *predict* a wonderful treat, toy, or tactile reward. If the patient's stress level is increasing, stop and reassess the situation. Done properly, desensitization should not elicit a stress response.

Example exposure ladder for subcutaneous injection:

- Patient remains stationary while approached, or chooses to approach veterinary team member, establishing a nonstressful starting point
- Reach toward a nonsensitive area near the injection site
- Glide toward the injection site

- Pick up the syringe in your other hand, and reach toward the nonsensitive area
- Glide toward the injection site
- Touch the injection site lightly
- Tent the skin slightly
- Tent the skin to the degree required for injection
- Approach the tented skin with the capped syringe
- Approach the tented skin with the capped syringe, and pinch the skin mildly
- With the capped syringe near the skin tent, pinch firmly to simulate a needle stick
- Touch the capped syringe softly to the injection site
- Touch the capped syringe firmly to the injection site
- Remove the syringe cap, and perform the handling steps
- Administer injection.

Figure 6.7 shows a diagram of this exposure ladder. Table 6.4 provides a worksheet example for one training session using desensitization and counterconditioning for injections.

Video 6.4 shows a puppy who has previously been a Level One patient for her earlier vaccinations. During this visit, she is eating treats as a distraction to prepare for her injection. When the technician touches the injection site, the puppy flinches and jumps slightly, showing an increase in stress in anticipation of the needle stick. The technician changes tactics, breaking the injection process down into several approximations, including tenting the skin, pinching the skin, and then injecting once the puppy seems relaxed again. Notice the client's response: amazement that the puppy tolerated the injection. This procedure took only a few seconds, but improved the puppy's experience considerably.

Video 6.5 shows a complete desensitization and classical conditioning start-to-finish for a cat to subcutaneous injections.

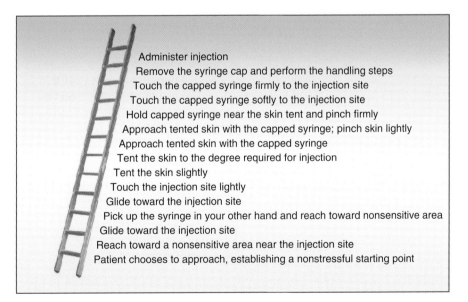

Figure 6.7 Example exposure ladder for injection training.

Table 6.4 Desensitization and counterconditioning worksheet for subcutaneous injection.

Training plan: Desensitization and counterconditioning	
Trigger: Subcutaneous injection, owner needs to begin giving insulin at home Session 1	Exposure ladder: Choose to approach; allow contact Reach toward nonsensitive area Glide to injection site Repeat steps, with syringe in hand
Foundation behaviors required: Orient/attention to team member Station helpful but not required	Touching of injection site Tenting skin at injection site Approach with syringe Tap skin with capped syringe Simulate injection while pinching skin Handling steps and pinch Actual injection
Preferred rewards to generate positive emotional response 1. Baby food 2. Canned cat food 3. Tactile of cheeks	
Medications: None required	Working area: Exam room 3, owner's lap
Nonstressful starting point: Patient sitting in owner's lap soliciting for treats	
Distance	Close proximity throughout procedure. No change when syringe is closer to patient.
Duration	Initial interactions 2–3 seconds, simulated injection ~5 seconds, actual injection ~1 second
Pressure	Starting pressure light petting, gradually worked up to strong pinch, and finally actual injection. Pinch was noticed more than the injection.
Volume	N/A
Other	Patient comfortable with complete progression of touch. Repeated the capped syringe injection twice when cat did not show interest in food after the first attempt. Interest in food returned for the next approximation.
Endpoint	Injection
Homework	Administer first 3 days of insulin injections using the full progression shown today. This should take about 60 seconds per injection. Then over the next 3 days, begin shortening the process so the final behavior is prepare injection, patient shows up, touch, glide, pinch, inject for a total time of about 15–30 seconds.
Plan for next visit	None needed unless questions; complete DS/CC protocol completed during first visit

In both video examples, notice the patient is comfortable with the process and no restraint is required. By taking a few extra seconds or minutes, one person can accomplish a task that may have previously required two or three team members.

Video 6.6 shows a mixed-breed dog, Kylie. This dog will always need sedation for certain procedures but has successfully learned how to accept restraint and intramuscular injection using desensitization and classical counterconditioning. Notice how Alicea breaks the behavior into small training steps, making sure the exposure ladder has enough rungs to keep Kiley calm enough to participate.

Venipuncture

Cephalic

Cephalic venipuncture for Level Two patients uses desensitization and classical conditioning to walk the pet through the process without restraint, and without causing an increase in fear or stress. With blood collection, each step in the desensitization process should predict something wonderful. Sometimes, it makes sense to allow the animal to keep eating throughout the process, while other patients will do better with the touch–treat–touch–treat rhythm. Don't be afraid to experiment and see which method works best for a specific patient.

As always, the technician providing the treats and support or stabilization will be monitoring the animal's body language throughout the procedure, and alerting the person collecting blood to any important changes or the need for a pause and regroup. If the animal struggles or tries to move away, stop, and add more rungs to the exposure ladder. Also, with peripheral venipuncture in general, butterfly catheters can make unrestrained procedures easier, because a small patient movement will not spoil the sample collection.

A sample exposure ladder for cephalic venipuncture could look like:

- Allow one technician to approach and feed; nonstressful starting point
- Technician with food reaches over or under and provides a stabilizing hand in case of unexpected responses from the patient
  - Break down into reaching over and touching as 2–3 steps, if needed
- Technician collecting blood approaches
- Touch the limb where blood will be collected at the shoulder
  - Glide touch to the elbow
- Use hand touching elbow to apply a "hand tourniquet" lightly
  - (Other tourniquets require adding rungs to the ladder here)
- Occlude the vessel
  - Only pick up the limb if the patient offers it; otherwise, leave it in a natural position
- Palpate
- Apply alcohol
- Approach with syringe
- Mimic venipuncture with capped syringe
- Pinch the area with a fingernail to assess response to sharp stimulus
- Collect blood
- Apply pressure or bandage after venipuncture is complete

Video 6.7 shows desensitization and counterconditioning to cephalic venipuncture with Reagan, a Flat-coated retriever. One technician offers food and helps the dog remain stationary, while the second collects blood. The technician collecting blood gradually goes through the steps in the exposure ladder, making sure to approach from a non-threatening position just below the patient. At one point, the dog pauses eating and notes what the technician is doing. She is only checking to see what is going on. The rest of her body language is relaxed. After checking in, she immediately returns to eating, and the sample is easily collected.

Lateral Saphenous (Dogs)

For Level Two dogs, consider the use of a butterfly catheter as previously mentioned. One technician will stabilize the patient and provide the food, while a second collects the sample. For very large dogs, a third person may be needed to help stabilize the dog's rear, as demonstrated for Level One dogs.

Sample exposure ladder for lateral saphenous blood collection:

- Dog stands comfortably and does not move away when technician approaches, establishing a nonstressful starting point
- Technician stabilizes the dog and pets the neck in case of unexpected responses
- Second technician touches the hip
- Glide hand down to stifle
- Glide hand to back of stifle
- Apply mild pressure where vein will be occluded
- Occlude the vessel
- Touch the injection area
- Apply alcohol
- Touch the area firmly
- Touch firmly with capped needle, or pinch to assess response to sharp stimulus
- Perform venipuncture
- Apply pressure or bandage after venipuncture is complete.

Figure 6.8 illustrates an exposure ladder for venipuncture. Video 6.8 features Mufasa, a Greyhound who is moderately stressed. The team attempts to collect the blood using a distraction technique, but the dog can't eat even high-value hot dogs while the setup for blood collection is done. After consulting the owner, the technician changes the treats to canned dog food. While one technician feeds and offers stabilizing neck scratches to establish a nonstressful starting point, the second gently moves through the exposure ladder for venipuncture. The dog pauses eating briefly in response to a noise from another room, then relaxes and returns to eating while venipuncture is performed.

Medial Saphenous (Cats)

Level Two cats are still relaxed enough to allow support and gentle manipulations, and accept food and/or tactile rewards intermittently during handling (Figure 6.9). For medial saphenous collection, the positioning is the same as for Level One, with the cat sternal or voluntarily lateral, lying on a hip with the back legs extended. For Level Two cats, progress through each step of the blood collection in a gradual fashion, with each step predicting something the cat enjoys such as a treat or facial petting. It is sometimes helpful to have a third person available to offer treats during this process.

Example exposure ladder for medial saphenous blood collection:

- Cat allows gentle positioning into a down position, establishing a nonstressful starting point
- One technician gently stabilizes the head

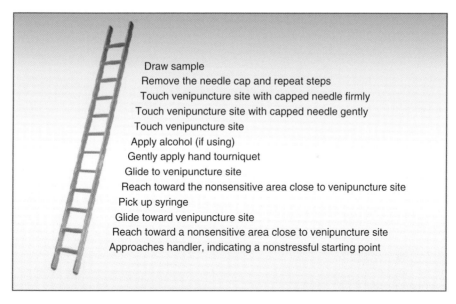

Draw sample
Remove the needle cap and repeat steps
Touch venipuncture site with capped needle firmly
Touch venipuncture site with capped needle gently
Touch venipuncture site
Apply alcohol (if using)
Gently apply hand tourniquet
Glide to venipuncture site
Reach toward the nonsensitive area close to venipuncture site
Pick up syringe
Glide toward venipuncture site
Reach toward a nonsensitive area close to venipuncture site
Approaches handler, indicating a nonstressful starting point

Figure 6.8 Example exposure ladder for venipuncture.

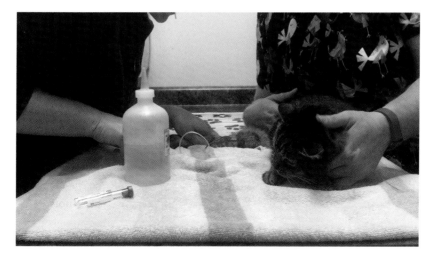

Figure 6.9 Positioning for medial saphenous blood collection with a Level Two feline patient.

- Occlude vessel gently with only the necessary pressure to raise a vein
- Second technician strokes the inner thigh
- Touch the venipuncture site
- Apply alcohol
- Palpate the vein
- Use a capped syringe or butterfly to simulate injection
- Pinch the venipuncture site firmly to simulate a sharp sensation
- Perform venipuncture
- Apply pressure or a bandage to the venipuncture site.

Video 6.9 demonstrates this technique with a Level Two feline patient. Notice the good communication between the team members, and the attentiveness to the patient's stress levels.

Jugular

Dogs are better candidates for desensitization and counterconditioning to jugular venipuncture than cats, because the positioning is more natural. Level Two dogs are likely to prefer to stand or sit, while Level Two cats will usually prefer to lie down with their paws retracted. It is easy to collect jugular blood from a dog who is standing or sitting, but challenging to collect from a cat who wants to lie sternally with her paws pulled in.

Example exposure ladder for jugular blood collection for dogs:

- Dog approaches handler or allows handler to approach, establishing a nonstressful starting point
- Handler gently touches under chin
- Handler raises chin slightly
- Technician collecting blood approaches
- Stroke between the front legs
- Glide up to the thoracic inlet
- Lightly touch the jugular furrow
- Occlude the vessel
- Palpate the vessel with the opposite hand
- Pinch the skin to simulate a sharp stimulus
- Simulate blood collection with a capped needle
- Perform venipuncture
- Apply pressure to the venipuncture site.

 Video 6.10 demonstrates the timing for desensitization for jugular blood collection. When compared to the distraction technique video in Level One, you will notice that the timing of the food is different. For this dog, each step in the process *predicts* a great treat, rather than using the food as a distraction throughout the process.

Blood Pressure Measurement

We should question the validity of the test results for blood pressure measurements when a patient is showing Level Two signs of mild to moderate stress and anxiety. While desensitization and counterconditioning to this procedure are relatively simple, if the patient is nervous enough to require desensitization, the test results will likely be inaccurate. For patients who will require serial blood pressure measurements, DS/CC is likely worthwhile. For a single measurement, anxiety-reducing medications can be considered prior to the measurement.

Example desensitization exposure ladder for blood pressure measurement:

- Patient approaches handler, or allows handler to approach without moving away, establishing a nonstressful starting point
- With the patient in a natural position, select the limb to be used
- Begin touch of the limb high on the leg at the shoulder or hip
- Glide to the next distal joint
- Glide to the area where the cuff will be applied

- Approach with the cuff; allow animal to investigate if they show interest
- Touch the limb with the cuff
- Wrap the cuff halfway around the limb
- Close the cuff around the limb
- Glide touch to the paw
- Touch the artery
- Using plenty of gel placed on the crystal, approach the paw
- Touch the crystal lightly to the paw
- Hold the crystal to the paw, and acquire the signal using headphones
- Inflate the cuff one-half pump
- Deflate the cuff
- Inflate the cuff one full pump
- Deflate the cuff
- Inflate the cuff until the signal is ceased
- Measure Doppler blood pressure
- Use a paper towel to remove the crystal and wipe away any gel
- Remove the cuff, minimizing Velcro closure sounds.

Cystocentesis

Cystocentesis is a procedure that can have very rare but serious adverse events associated if the patient is too tense or moves too much during the puncture. To avoid these unwanted outcomes (e.g., laceration or rupture of the bladder, peritonitis, vasovagal response, abdominal vessel perforation, and GI injury), help patients be as comfortable as possible during this procedure.[1-3] For Level Two dogs and cats, consider providing medical management of anxiety, and then following the procedures described for Level One patients. If the patient is still too nervous to participate without excessive stress and struggling, sedation should be provided, or a sterile free-catch sample considered.

6.6 Administering Medications and Grooming

Medication Stations

Level Two patients can benefit from medication stations just as Level One patients can. The medication station is a powerful tool, because it allows the patient to give consent for the procedure by remaining at the station, and withdraw consent simply by leaving. Because so many rewards are given to reinforce the stationing behavior, the patient should have a highly positive emotional response to being at the station. This positive emotional response helps to establish a nonstressful starting point for desensitization and classical counterconditioning for Level Two pets.

Oral Medications

Level Two dogs are not comfortable being held to manually give a pill. When provided with a pill wrapped in a treat, they will often find the pill, eating around it and spitting out or avoiding ingesting the pill. These patients will quickly learn they are only being given a certain special food when it contains a pill, and will begin to avoid that special food entirely because it predicts a "sour berry" if we revisit the analogy from Chapter 5. When oral medications are prescribed, provide the client with enough education to successfully administer the medications at home, and make sure the client understands to call the clinic for help if there are problems giving the medication.

To administer a pill, use treats the animal receives at other times, such as for training and during medication time. Have at least five total treats, one containing the pill. Invite the patient to the medication station. Click and treat rapidly and repeatedly for the stationing behavior, using the pill treat as one of these rewards. When these patients go into "training mode" mentally, they will often be more focused on the task at hand than on investigating the treats for concealed pills. If the patient is not trained for a medication station, ask for a group of other trained behaviors or tricks, such as sit, down, shake, spin, or any other tricks the patient knows. Click and treat for each trick, with the pill treat being one of the ones used during the clicking and treating session. Another approach is to use the meatball-to-meal method. Instruct clients to prepare the animal's meal, making a production of the event. Then, a pill should be concealed in a meatball of canned pet food or sticky treats. Hold the meatball in one hand, and the meal in the other. Give the meatball, and as the pet is swallowing the meatball, immediately follow by offering the remainder of the meal.

For liquid medications, the same guidelines apply. Prepare the liquid medication as described in Chapter 5, and then use the syringes to administer treats when clicking and treating at the medication station or in response to cued behaviors. Either hold both syringes and rotate the medicine syringe into the mix, or set the syringe down each time, changing which syringe is picked up so that the patient receives a few plain treats from a syringe, then the medicine treat, then a few more plain treats to finish up.

For particularly discerning patients, compounding medications is a great option. Many medicines can be made into a flavored liquid or a flavored chewable treat to at least partly disguise the medication. Some medicines may not make a good liquid or chewable treat, but can be compounded into a capsule that is at least flavorless on the outside, and has no medicine taste unless the capsule is bitten and punctured. Keeping some plain gel capsules in the clinic to dispense with bitter medications such as metronidazole and tramadol can ease administration. The pill or fragment can be placed inside the gel capsule by the owner prior to administration. It is important not to handle the gel capsule if there is powder from the pill on your hands, as this will flavor the outside of the capsule, defeating the purpose of decreasing the unpleasant taste.

Ear Medications and Cleaning

Level Two patients may start out allowing ear cleansing and medications with distractions, but may escalate, become nervous, stop eating, or try to move away even though food is being offered. These patients will benefit from desensitization and classical counterconditioning to break down the process and help build a positive cooperative response. If the animal has a painful ear, pain medication should be provided prior to working with the ear, and applying a topical anesthetic cream to the pinna and external ear canal can make the procedure more comfortable. This product should *not* be inserted deep into the ear.

Break down the ear-cleansing and ear-medicating process into an exposure ladder, making sure to find a nonstressful or least-stressful starting point. Each step on the exposure ladder should predict wonderful treats, and the patient needs to be comfortable enough to eat for each approximation. Monitor food acceptance, body language, and proximity preference throughout the procedure. If the patient's stress level is increasing, try adding more rungs to the exposure ladder, breaking the process into smaller steps. If that does not help, stop the procedure, and provide improved medical management of pain, stress, and anxiety prior to continuing. Please do not add assistants restraining the patient to the mix. If it takes two or more people to physically restrain a patient for any kind of treatment, we are doing harm to that patient, and need to stop and make a new plan.

Example exposure ladder for ear medication:

- The patient approaches, or remains still while approached, establishing a nonstressful starting point
- Touch a less sensitive area, such as the shoulder
- Glide toward the ear
- Touch the base of the ear
- Touch the pinna lightly
- Place a finger and thumb on either side of the pinna, preparing to position it
- Pick up ear medication, swab, or the like
- Touch a less sensitive area
- Glide toward the ear
- Touch the base of the ear
- Touch the pinna lightly
- Place a finger and thumb on either side of the pinna, preparing to position it
- Touch the ear canal opening with a finger
- Move the medicine vial closer to the patient: this may require several incremental movements
- Touch the medicine vial to the ear
- Insert the medicine applicator into the ear
- Dispense medication
- Massage the ear canal to distribute medication
- Touch a less sensitive area to finish.

Table 6.5 is an example of a possible worksheet from a desensitization and counterconditioning session for ear cleansing. Figure 6.10 shows a possible exposure ladder for ear treatment.

Training Tip: Touch It

If there is an existing negative response to a piece of equipment such as nail trimmers, the ear cleanser bottle, or eye drops, considering using the object for a game of targeting. Use shaping to encourage the patient to target the object with a nose or a paw, and reward frequently for this behavior. Making a game out of interacting with potentially scary items can decrease fear and improve conditioned emotional responses as well.

Table 6.5 Desensitization and counterconditioning worksheet for ear cleansing.

Training plan: Desensitization and counterconditioning	
Trigger: Ear cleansing, routine Owner needs to clean ears at home for maintenance and grooming Session 2	Exposure ladder: Patient chooses to approach Touch nonsensitive area Glide to ear Short duration touch, longer duration Hold ear cleanser and repeat steps
Foundation behaviors required: Approach/attend handler Station helpful but not required	Touch ear Base, mid, pinna, lift/open Touch with dry cotton ball Touch with wet cotton ball brief Increase duration with wet cotton ball Cleanse ear
Preferred rewards to generate positive emotional response 1. Bacon 2. Cheese 3. Tennis ball	
Medications: None required	Working area: Exam room 1, mat on floor
Nonstressful starting point: Dog approaches handler and chooses to interact	
Distance	Patient comfortable with close proximity
Duration	Began with 1–2 seconds of ear handling with dry cotton. Gradually progress to 15 seconds of swabbing and massage with dry cotton.
Pressure	Started with a gliding touch, progressed to firm massage with fingers and cotton.
Volume	N/A
Other	Progression through exposure ladder was cautious and gradual. Endpoint during session 1 was approaching with dry cotton; patient tolerated this within two approximations and made significant progress.
Endpoint	Dry cotton tactile for 15 seconds; external manual massage of ear canal
Homework	Dry cotton tactile for 15 seconds; external massage of ear canal
Plan for next visit	Increase from dry cotton to wet cotton tactile for 15–30 seconds

Remember: if the animal has a decrease in food acceptance, shows more stress markers in his body language, or tries to move away, it does not mean the method is ineffective. Allow him to opt out and take a break when needed, and watch for him to return and show he is ready to try again. He is simply giving us great information about what he needs: more rungs on the exposure ladder, more medical management, different treats, a break from training, or to be moved to a Level Three training protocol as described in Chapter 7.

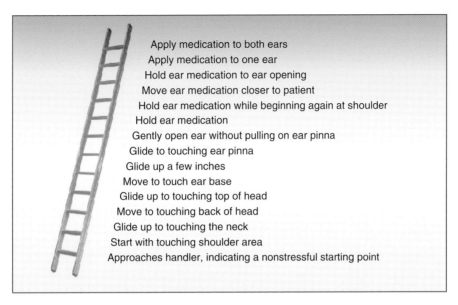

Apply medication to both ears
Apply medication to one ear
Hold ear medication to ear opening
Move ear medication closer to patient
Hold ear medication while beginning again at shoulder
Hold ear medication
Gently open ear without pulling on ear pinna
Glide to touching ear pinna
Glide up a few inches
Move to touch ear base
Glide up to touching top of head
Move to touching back of head
Glide up to touching the neck
Start with touching shoulder area
Approaches handler, indicating a nonstressful starting point

Figure 6.10 Exposure ladder example for ear treatment.

Video 6.11 shows the desensitization and counterconditioning process for applying ear medication with Dresdan. Notice he approaches the handlers, and is unrestrained. The choice to stay or to opt out is his, establishing a point of consent for the procedure. As each approximation is completed, a delicious food reward is provided to improve the emotional response and also to try to reinforce the behavior of remaining still and participating in ear treatment.

Eye Medications

For patients who will need lifelong eye drops, such as those with dry eye, allergies, or glaucoma, consider Level Three training as described in Chapter 7. For Level Two patients, desensitization and counterconditioning should be sufficient. Use regular saline or a plain eye rinse for the training period, then move to medicated drops when appropriate (Figure 6.11).

Example exposure ladder for eye drops:

- Patient approaches or does not move away when approached, establishing a non-stressful starting point
- Touch a less sensitive area, such as the shoulder or dorsal neck
- Glide toward the head, avoiding the ear
- Glide toward the upper eyelid
- Pick up the saline drop bottle
- Touch a less sensitive area
- Glide toward the head, avoiding the ear
- Glide toward the upper eyelid
- Touch just above the upper eyelid
- Apply light pressure just above the upper eyelid, as if to hold the eye open

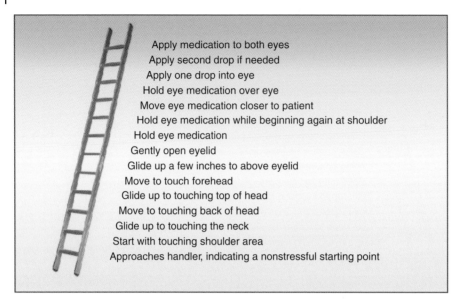

Apply medication to both eyes
Apply second drop if needed
Apply one drop into eye
Hold eye medication over eye
Move eye medication closer to patient
Hold eye medication while beginning again at shoulder
Hold eye medication
Gently open eyelid
Glide up a few inches to above eyelid
Move to touch forehead
Glide up to touching top of head
Move to touching back of head
Glide up to touching the neck
Start with touching shoulder area
Approaches handler, indicating a nonstressful starting point

Figure 6.11 Exposure ladder example for eye treatment.

- Approach with the saline drops
- Hold the saline drops over the head
- Dispense a drop onto the fur of the head or muzzle, *not* into the eye
- Repeat the drop-dispensing step until the patient is comfortable with a few locations
- Place a drop into the eye
- Finish by touching a less sensitive area
- Repeat, using actual eye medication.

 Video 6.12 shows rapid desensitization and classical counterconditioning to eye drops with Kanga. Notice she is allowed to move away if she chooses to do so, and every repetition predicts a treat. The exposure ladder is designed to create a touching routine that shows the dog we are going to administer eye drops. The drops are never a surprise, and she is allowed to become comfortable with drops in alternate locations before a drop actually lands in her eye.

Training Tip: Harness the Power of Medication Stations

Pets who understand the medication station will love to visit it. It is an antecedent for fun, treats, and handling games. We can use the positive emotions and excitement linked with the medication station to encourage patients to enjoy treatments like eye drops. Remember to maintain fun at the medication station, so the patient trusts it and finds experiences there to be predictably pleasant.

Nail Trims

Many patients have a negative emotional association with nail trimming. This could be due to personal preference; increased sensitivity of the paws (natural differences or due to illness); history of fear-provoking nail trims involving excessive restraint; history of nails trimmed too short, causing pain; or nail trims during another stressful event (e.g., a dog is barking in another room), causing a lasting emotional impression. As discussed in Chapter 5, grooming is never a good reason to permanently damage the relationship between the veterinary team and the patient, poison the veterinary clinic as a good place, or put team members and the patient at risk for injury. More restraint is not the right answer for grooming. Train the pet, instead!

Level Two nail trim patients are reluctant to take food as a distraction, or stop eating when they are touched, but do not show any defensive or aggressive behaviors. If the patient is showing defensive aggression, provide medical management and move to Level Three training techniques.

Example exposure ladder for nail trims (this example is for a front paw, but can be adapted for rear paws as well) (Figure 6.12):

- Patient approaches technician, or chooses not to move away when approached, establishing a nonstressful starting point
- Touch a nonsensitive area, such as the shoulder
- Glide toward the elbow
- Glide toward the carpus/wrist
- Glide toward the paw
- Lift the paw an inch*
  - Gradually lift the paw higher with each approximation until a comfortable height for clipping
  - * Some patients' conformation allows nail clipping without raising the paw
- Pick up the nail trimmers
- Touch the shoulder

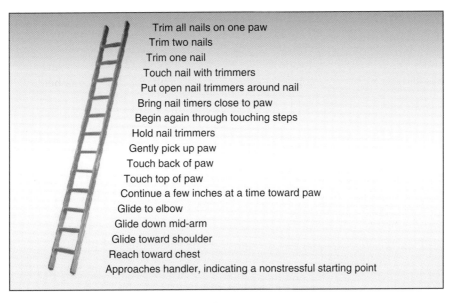

Trim all nails on one paw
Trim two nails
Trim one nail
Touch nail with trimmers
Put open nail trimmers around nail
Bring nail timers close to paw
Begin again through touching steps
Hold nail trimmers
Gently pick up paw
Touch back of paw
Touch top of paw
Continue a few inches at a time toward paw
Glide to elbow
Glide down mid-arm
Glide toward shoulder
Reach toward chest
Approaches handler, indicating a nonstressful starting point

Figure 6.12 Exposure ladder example for nail trimming.

- Glide toward the elbow, then the carpus
- Glide toward the paw
- Lift the paw a small distance
- Lift to comfortable nail trim height
- Isolate a toe
  - Hold the toe for 1 second
  - Gradually hold the toe for longer periods of time
- Approach the toenail with clippers
- Surround the toenail with clipper
- Tap the toenail, making a clicking sound
- Clip one toenail
- Clip multiple toenails
- Finish by touching a less sensitive area.

Table 6.6 shows a worksheet example for a desensitization and counterconditioning session for nail trimming.

For some patients, this process can be accomplished by one person in less than 1 minute. For other patients, the process can take several visits, even with anxiety-reducing medications. Remember: grooming is virtually never an emergency need, and if it is, simply use sedation rather than risking lasting emotional trauma to the animal.

Video 6.13 shows a technician working solo with Shelby, a Labrador who has uncomfortable feet due to allergies. This dog is invited to participate in nail trimming, and a short DS/CC protocol is used to successfully trim one, and then all the nails. Observe the dog's body language. She shifts between relaxed and mild stress. She chooses to move away at times, but is unrestrained and repeatedly opts into the training process on her own. This nail trim took 4 minutes for one team member. The second clip shows Shelby's next visit. Notice the toenail trim goes much quicker, and the dog is even more relaxed.

Anal Gland Expression

Anal gland expression is an invasive procedure. Many patients are fearful for this procedure, and those who aren't initially, often become so. Using a topical anesthetic cream can help ease the process, decreasing tactile sensitivity for the patient. For this example, one person stabilizes the dog, while another expresses the anal glands.

Example exposure ladder for anal gland expression (Figure 6.13):

- Patient does not move away when technician approaches from the side, establishing a nonstressful starting point
- Technician reaches in front to stabilize the patient
- Technician reaches across the patient's body
- Technician begins stabilizing the patient
- Second technician approaches from the side
- Touch a less sensitive area, such as the dorsal rump, lateral thigh, or hip
- Glide toward the rectal area
- Place a hand between the tail and the rectum
- Use a flat hand to raise the tail without grasping it
- Apply anesthetic cream or jelly

Table 6.6 Desensitization and counterconditioning worksheet for nail trims.

Training plan: Desensitization and counterconditioning	
Trigger: Nail trim Session 3	Exposure ladder: Session 3: Orient and allow approach
Foundation behaviors required: Orient to handler Stationing helpful but not required	Paw lift starting at shoulder Touch trimmer to nail Make noise of trimmer near nail Encircle nail with trimmer Tap nail with trimmer Clip one nail
Preferred rewards to generate positive emotional response 1. Steak 2. Chicken 3. Cheese	
Medications: Alprazolam night before and 2 hours prior	Working area: Rubber mats Exam Room 3
Nonstressful starting point: Orient to handler on rubber mats, allow shoulder touch	
Distance	Nail trimmer distance was 12" from front paw, gradual approach until contact with nail
Duration	Initial duration: 10 seconds per touch; final duration: 10 seconds, including trimming one nail
Pressure	Initial pressure was no contact, gradual increase to tapping, pressing, and clipping nail
Volume	Sound of nail clippers introduced when clippers were 6" away, then gradually closer to increase sound influence
Other	Tactile increase from no contact gradually up to trimming one front nail
Endpoint	Trimming one front toenail
Homework	Trim front nails one at a time
Plan for next visit	Begin training for rear paws

- Palpate the rectal area lightly
- Touch the anus with a finger lubricated with anesthetic gel
- Insert the finger; palpate the gland
- Express the gland
- Reposition for the second gland
- Palpate
- Express
- Cleanse the area with a damp paper towel and odor-reducing product.

When possible, work with the owner present. Owners often underestimate how invasive some pets perceive this procedure to be, and the skill level of the technicians

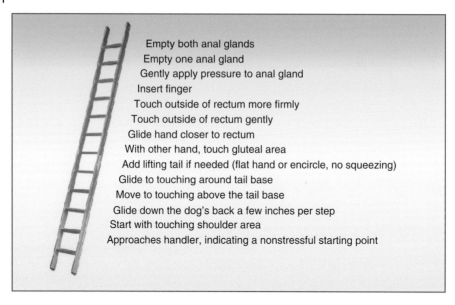

Empty both anal glands
Empty one anal gland
Gently apply pressure to anal gland
Insert finger
Touch outside of rectum more firmly
Touch outside of rectum gently
Glide hand closer to rectum
With other hand, touch gluteal area
Add lifting tail if needed (flat hand or encircle, no squeezing)
Glide to touching around tail base
Move to touching above the tail base
Glide down the dog's back a few inches per step
Start with touching shoulder area
Approaches handler, indicating a nonstressful starting point

Figure 6.13 Exposure ladder example for anal gland expression.

performing the procedure. If the patient shows increasing signs of stress and is struggling, pause the procedure and consider a new plan.

Video 6.14 shows two technicians attempting an anal gland expression using the distraction technique. This technique is not appropriate for the patient, as he turns toward the technician, becomes more nervous, and shows avoidance behaviors. The technicians change to a desensitization and counterconditioning protocol, where each touch and step in the process predict food. The technicians communicate with one another about when to give food, and when to withhold it. If no touching is being done, no food is given. By breaking the procedure into multiple approximations and teaching the dog that each step *predicts* something good, the procedure was completed in a single visit.

Conclusion

Level Two patients are generally more anxious and concerned about veterinary care. These patients may become wary during distraction techniques, or avoid handling when the progression of handling is too fast. Using systematic desensitization and classical conditioning or counterconditioning improves patient care. Remember: training is a patient-directed process. The patient is allowed to opt in or opt out of training, and the desensitization and counterconditioning process should look boring or happy, rather than increasing the patient's stress level. If the patient opts out, rewind the process to a nonstressful point, and begin again, adding more rungs to the exposure ladder; or stop training for the day and try again when the patient is more relaxed, using even smaller baby steps during the next session. By empowering our patients to direct their treatment plans, we can earn lasting trust and provide a higher standard of care. When we show empathy for patient stress and make efforts to reduce it, the veterinary care experience is improved for patient, client, and the entire veterinary team.

References

1 Brown, C. (2006) Diagnostic cystocentesis: Techniques and considerations. *Lab Animal*. 35 (4), 21–23.
2 Buckley, G. (2009). Massive transfusion and surgical management of iatrogenic aortic laceration associated with cystocentesis in a dog. *Journal of the American Veterinary Medical Association*. 235 (3), 288–291.
3 Odunayo, A., *et al.* (2015) Probable vasovagal reaction following cystocentesis in two cats. *Journal of Feline Medicine and Surgery Open Reports*. 1 (1), 1–4. doi:10.1177/2055116915585021.
4 Forterre, F., *et al.* (2007) Iatrogenic sciatic nerve injury in eighteen dogs and nine cats. *Veterinary Surgery*. 36 (5), 464–471.

7

Level Three Patients and Training

7.1 Level Three Training

Level Three training has many applications. Level Three methods should be considered for any patient, but they require a time investment and some training skills for success. Some clients, especially if they are sophisticated trainers, may express interest in learning Level Three skills even for relaxed, cooperative patients. These owners are highly motivated to build great experiences for their pets.

Relying on a combination of desensitization and classical conditioning paired with operant conditioning, Level Three training establishes a language of consent for the patients while conditioning them to accept and even enjoy care. Remember to take the time to set up the environment to be as nonstressful as possible, and review the medical record for success notes and individual preferences before you begin.

Patients who assess at Level Three may have unwanted behaviors in the veterinary clinic due to negative past experiences, intrinsic fears, or a combination of both. Level Three dogs and cats are experiencing severe emotional distress. These patients require intervention to try to reverse the fear response, and then instruct the patient how to cooperate for care.

When working with Level Three patients, use the same patient evaluation tool as for Level One and Level Two (Figure 7.1). Unless the patient has a true need for immediate veterinary care, Level Three patients should be slated for medical management, training visits, and attempting care once these services have been offered. Training visits can be provided by technicians, veterinarians, or trainers who are comfortable with the techniques and skilled in the application of desensitization, classical conditioning, and operant conditioning. Sometimes, as few as 1–3 visits are required, while in other circumstances five or more preparatory visits are needed. The client should be counseled in advance about the anticipated time required for training, the costs associated, and how to build realistic expectations. In general, the more fearful the patient is during initial assessment, the longer the training process will take.

The time investment for Level Three training may seem overwhelming for some owners. A few owners may be hesitant to invest the time and money required to achieve the goal of training all behaviors, including full examination, sample collection, and so on. It might not take as much time as the owner thinks. Once an animal has learned to train for their first voluntary behavior, subsequent behaviors are easier to train because the animal understands the process. For owners with Level Three patients who consider

Cooperative Veterinary Care, First Edition. Alicea Howell and Monique Feyrecilde.
© 2018 John Wiley & Sons, Inc. Published 2018 by John Wiley & Sons, Inc.
Companion website: www.wiley.com/go/howell/cooperative

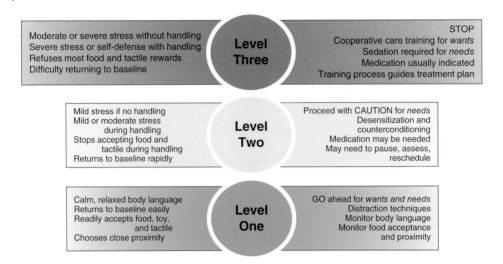

Figure 7.1 Assessment of Level Three patients.

their options and still decide they don't wish to pursue full cooperative procedure training, teaching the dog or cat to allow low-stress sedation protocols will be a realistic goal. Many of these techniques mirror the handling methods used for wild animals housed in zoos and aquaria. How would we obtain blood from a killer whale? How many people would be required to manually restrain the animal? Would sedation be appropriate and safe? The answer: we collect blood from a killer whale by training cooperative husbandry and veterinary care behaviors. If a goldfish can learn agility, or a shark can cooperate for abdominal ultrasound, a dog or cat can certainly learn to cooperate for physical examination, blood collection, and injections with the proper training.

Training Tip: Life in a Perfect World

In a perfect world, Level Three training would be the option selected for every patient, because it allows complete voluntary and cooperative care. The patient directs how care is administered, and the veterinary team communicates clearly and respectfully what the animal needs to do to be successful.

7.2 Identifying Level Three Patients

As mentioned, some Level Three patients are calm and cooperative, but have owners who are interested in less invasive and better trained veterinary care. The remainder are those who are too fearful to permit care without medical management and training. The goal with Level Three patients is to lower their stress levels to the point where they can constructively learn new skills, and then train the necessary skills to allow care. Level Three patients may display some or all of these signs. As with Level One and Level Two, we need to be flexible and monitor the patient continuously. Many patients will display aspects of Level Two and Level Three during the same assessment. ***Even one Level Three marker is enough to score a patient as Level Three.***

Level Three Dogs

Food Acceptance
- Dogs will accept food from the owner or pick it up off the floor, or may refuse all food
- Will not accept high-value food from most or all team members
- Rarely may accept high-value food from trusted team members
- Takes food with a hard mouth, even when not being handled
- May take food quickly, then retreat ("snakebite")
- If accepting some food at any point, food acceptance stops during any handling attempts
- Difficulty returning to baseline food acceptance, even from the owner, after handling attempts

Body Language
- Mild, moderate, or severe stress body language in the hospital when not being handled (refer to Chapter 2)
- May show moderate and severe stress markers during handling:
  - Dilated pupils with widened eyes; sclera may be visible
  - Scanning the environment; hypervigilance
  - Increased respiratory rate; possible stress panting
  - Ears held flat or pulled back
  - Tail held low or tucked up against the abdomen
  - Piloerection
  - Tries to escape when handling attempted
  - May freeze when handling attempted
  - Possible defensive aggression during handling attempts
  - Vocalization
  - Possible signs of learned helplessness
- When the handling and procedure are stopped, difficulty returning to baseline

Proximity Preference
- Off-leash, dog chooses to stay near the owner or hide (e.g., under a chair)
- Looks away and leans away when team members make social contact
- Will approach team members only for very high-value food or when the team member is looking and facing away
- Is reluctant or completely unable to come out from hiding places
- Actively tries to avoid or escape handling efforts

Table 7.1 is a quick reference checklist for assessing Level Three Dogs. Figure 7.2 depicts a Level Three Dog.

Level Three Cats

Level Three cats present unique challenges to the veterinary practitioner. Many owners of Level Three cats are unable to bring them to the veterinary clinic. Capturing the cat to place it in the carrier may be dangerous for the owner, because of defensive aggression. Also, the client's perception of stress may be so upsetting that the client avoids making appointments because they don't want their beloved pets to have such frightening experiences.

Table 7.1 Checklist for Level Three dogs: Each dog assessing at Level Three may have a combination of these attributes.

Stage of visit	Food acceptance	Body language	Proximity preference
Greeting	☐ Rarely accept food ☐ Will eat from floor but not from hand ☐ Hard mouth or rapid retreat	☐ Tense with mild, moderate, and/or severe stress markers	☐ Does not greet ☐ Hides ☐ May interact with owner
Touching	☐ Refuses food ☐ Difficulty returning to baseline	☐ Tense, fearful	☐ Avoidance ☐ Self-defense
Exam treatment	☐ Refuses food ☐ Difficulty returning to baseline	☐ Tense, fearful ☐ Difficulty returning to baseline	☐ Avoidance ☐ Self-defense ☐ Does not return to baseline

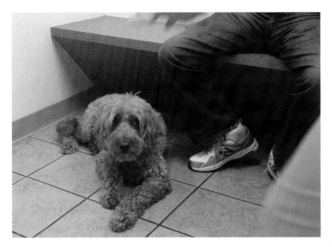

Figure 7.2 Level Three canine patient.

Because Level Three cats are in severe distress, and often the owner is very stressed as well, you will see more training for dogs than for cats in this chapter. The techniques used for dogs can be applied to cats, if the cat is in a good mental state for learning new skills. Most pet cats are more environmentally sensitive than dogs. Their social lives are considerably different. The expectations of skills and social experiences presented to dogs are much more varied than those presented to pet cats by most owners. The authors firmly believe cats are capable of learning to cooperate for veterinary behaviors! However, the unique challenges of the veterinary–client–patient relationship with cats and their owners make training cats in the veterinary clinic substantially more difficult. These methods can be applied in the home, via house calls, with the assistance of a veterinary behaviorist, or with the assistance of a skilled trainer.

Food Acceptance, Toy Acceptance, and Tactile Acceptance
- Does not investigate or accept food or toys
- May allow gentle petting/tactile by a team member for periods <3 seconds
- May allow petting by owner
- May or may not allow any petting/tactile

Body Language
Moderate or severe stress markers are present in the hospital.

- Moderate stress markers in the carrier or during handling attempts, such as:
  - Widened eyes with dilated pupils
  - Whiskers pulled forward; mouth tight
  - Ears held back or flat
  - Increased respiratory rate
  - Hypervigilant; scanning the environment
  - Tense muscles; flinches if touched
  - Tail tucked close to body or twitching/slashing
  - Piloerection
  - Vocalization
  - Defensive aggression
- Difficulty returning to baseline after handling attempts
- Difficulty returning to baseline after arriving home

Proximity Preference
- Chooses to hide in the carrier
- Chooses to exit the carrier, but hides elsewhere
- May explore exam room but cautiously, crouching or following walls
- Retreats when team members approach without attempting handling
- Moves away when handling is attempted
- Difficulty returning to baseline when handling attempts are ceased

Table 7.2 is a quick reference checklist for assessing Level Three cats. Figure 7.3 shows a Level Three Cat experiencing severe stress.

Table 7.2 Checklist for Level Three cats: Each cat assessing at Level Three may have a combination of these attributes.

Stage of visit	Food or tactile acceptance	Body language	Proximity preference
Greeting	☐ Refuses food ☐ Rarely allows brief tactile <3 seconds	☐ Tense with mild, moderate, and/or severe stress markers	☐ Hides in carrier ☐ May show self-defense when approached
Touching	☐ Refuses food and tactile ☐ Difficulty returning to baseline	☐ Tense, fearful	☐ Avoidance ☐ Self-defense
Exam treatment	☐ Refuses food and tactile ☐ Difficulty returning to baseline	☐ Tense, fearful ☐ Difficulty returning to baseline	☐ Avoidance ☐ Self-defense ☐ Does not return to baseline

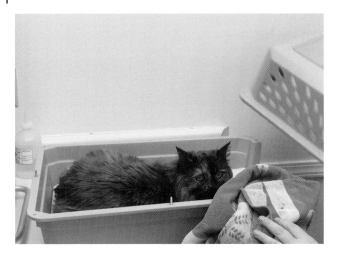

Figure 7.3 Level Three feline patient.

7.3 Preparing to Train

For Level Three training to work, the environment needs to be conducive to stress reduction and positive learning. Refer to Chapter 4 for ideas on setting up the examination room to maximize success. Level Three training should be done with the owner present in most cases. At first, the technician, veterinarian, or trainer (each are described as "trainer" in this chapter) should instruct the owner to ignore the patient during training sessions, but the eventual goal will likely include the owner's participation, and the owner may also be enlisted to do homework between sessions.

In some circumstances, the patient may be a candidate for Day Training, in which the pet is dropped off at the hospital for a series of training sessions throughout the day. Day Training candidates need to be relatively relaxed in the hospital environment for this strategy to succeed. Another option for some clients may be to cooperate with a qualified trainer outside the clinic, and with the help of the trainer, transition these skills to the clinic environment.

Make sure the appointment is scheduled to allow enough time. We suggest 30 minutes for initial appointments and 15 minutes for follow-ups. The client should be instructed to give all pre-visit medications at the correct interval, to fast the patient for at least six hours prior to the visit, and to come prepared with the patient's very favorite foods and toy.

Choose a room that can be set up the same way each time at first. Patients who are nervous in the hospital will be suspicious of change. Minimize change at first to maximize patient trust and comfort. Small changes to the environment can always be introduced later in the training process. After escorting the pet into the exam room, sit down and explain the goals of the training process to the owner. Does this patient need to cooperate for examination, vaccination, ear or eye care, or sample collection, or simply to allow sedation to go more smoothly? Invest a moment and discuss the plan and the goals with the client to assure everyone is on the same page (a phone interview prior to the visit can also serve this purpose). During this time, assess the patient's food acceptance, body language, and proximity preference while you're preparing to get started training. If the patient is too stressed to train, formulate a plan to improve the patient's response to the environment (home plan prior to transport, transport, environmental setup, medical management, etc.) prior to attempting Level Three training strategies.

The owner can be helpful by explaining what potential reinforcers they think the animal will like best, and what methods have been used in the past. Dogs who have been trained using punishment-based methods may be anticipating something unpleasant happening. Those who have been trained using lure-reward training may be waiting for a lure or treat to be presented prior to trying new skills. Level Three training relies heavily on shaping, and shaping requires the patient to be willing to explore the environment and try new things in an effort to earn clicks and treats. If the pet already has experience with shaping, training will progress more quickly. For patients who are new to shaping, we will first have to teach them the fun process of this game, and then how to apply the shaping process to acquiring new skills.

Establishing Consent and Operant Conditioning

Level Three training stresses voluntary, cooperative veterinary care. *Voluntary* means the animal is free to participate, or choose not to participate if they are feeling stressed. *Cooperative* means the patient understands to perform a certain behavior, or allow a specific touch, to earn a desired reward. To allow the animal to make this choice, the trainer needs to establish a consent point: a point at which the animal understands training will start and stop at his or her request. Level Three training is different because there is a **contingency** the animal must meet to earn a click and treat. For desensitization and counterconditioning, the animal received the food, toy, or tactile pleasant stimulus regardless of what they were doing. The goal was to create a conditioned positive emotional response. Level Three uses operant conditioning. The patient is learning to give consent and is opting in for training. The trainer can then begin requiring certain criteria to be met before a click and treat result.

The point of consent will be unique to each patient, and perhaps to each procedure. To communicate the idea of consent to the animal, the trainer will begin training when the desired consent point has occurred, and will immediately stop training if the consent behavior is withdrawn. By consistently starting and stopping training in this fashion, we can teach the animals how to control their own care and how to communicate if they are ready to continue or if they are feeling overwhelmed.

For example, we will use stationing as a consent point for some behaviors in this chapter. By choosing to go to the station, the patient is giving his consent to train for the procedure. To stop the session, the patient can simply move off the station (mat, table, rug, etc.). When the patient moves away from the station, all training, and therefore all reinforcement, stop (Figure 7.4). Any discomfort the patient may have been feeling during the training process will cease, but so will all the wonderful cookies and pleasant feedback associated with training. This cessation will both empower the patient to have more trust in the trainer, but also increase the value of the station and training. Hopefully, we will be encouraging the patient to feel good about the process, enjoy training, and be motivated to persist and continue. It is crucial that the trainer respect the point of consent for this method to work. The temptation for "one more repetition" or "I'm going to just put the drops in quickly" might be strong, especially as you near completion of a trained behavior. Remember: it takes only one bad experience to damage trust but many good experiences to gain it. Respect the point of consent, and retain the animal's trust.

(a)

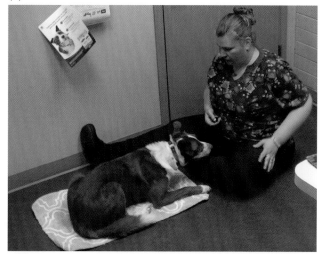

(b)

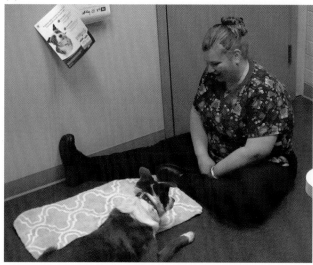

Figure 7.4 Canine patient choosing to move onto the station (a), and choosing to move off the station (b).

7.4 Making a Training Plan

Prior to starting training, get in the habit of making a training plan. The training plan is your roadmap to accomplishing the goal behavior. To make a simple veterinary procedure training plan, follow these steps:

1) Define the completed behavior.
   If there are multiple behaviors, each behavior needs its own smaller plan. For example, injections need a different plan from blood collection, which will both be separate from nail trims.

2) Determine the patient's preferred potential reinforcers. Identify at least three options, and rank them in order of preference.
3) Decide where to work.
4) Identify the point of consent.

There are a number of simple ways to establish consent points. Location is one method, such as choosing to move toward and stay on the station (mat, rug, and table). Another option is body position. If the procedure is to be done in a sitting position, the patient can withdraw consent by moving into a stand. Targeting, such as maintaining a chin rest or hand target, is another way to establish consent. The patient's preference, practicality of training, owner preference, and procedure to be performed will all dictate what the consent point will be. In some cases, each separate behavior may also have a separate point of consent.

5) Decide which foundation behaviors, if any, will be needed, and train foundation behaviors in advance.
6) Verify medications needed, if any.
7) Imagine approximations.

Shaping is all about *approximations*, or baby steps or building blocks toward a goal behavior (see Chapter 3 for a review of shaping techniques). Consider what the building blocks may be for your behavior, and then split them down as small as you can. The better you are at splitting behaviors into small approximations, the better you will be at shaping!

8) Establish criteria for reinforcement for approximations.
9) Determine advancement points where the patient is ready for criterion increases to earn reinforcers.
10) Plan to chart your progress using detailed notes or video.
11) Record the ending point for the training session.

Table 7.3 is an example training plan worksheet for Level Three training. In the Appendix, you will find training plan worksheets to help you build your own training plans. A few example training plans are included in this chapter to get you started. Remember: each patient is different, and will benefit from customizations to the training plan.

7.5 Getting Started: Approach, Target, and Station

We will be using mostly dog examples for these training videos, but remember: any animal can learn these behaviors with proper training and the right reinforcement.

Training Tip: Make a Movie
Videotape your training sessions. Reviewing the video will help you catch errors and improve your training skills. The videos are also excellent for tracking patient progress, and posting on social media.

Table 7.3 Level Three training plan worksheet: This is a basic template for the steps of creating a Level Three training plan.

Training plan: Level Three training	
Completed behavior:	Component behaviors:
Consent point:	Consent point:
Preferred reinforcers 1. 2. 3.	
Medications:	Working area:
Foundation behaviors required:	Known cues needed: Additional DS/CC/CC needed: Yes No
Starting criteria	
Progression	
Ending criteria	
Observations	
Homework	
Plan for next visit	

Available for download in the Online Resources.

Approaches

Every final veterinary behavior begins with the patient approaching a team member, and allowing some form of touch. Begin by training approaches. Once you're settled in the room, choose where you'd like the animal to work, such as a mat, rug, or low table. Sit or stand near the station. Watch the patient closely. At first, watch the patient's nose. The nose moving toward you will mean the dog is going to look at you, but the nose is often easier for you to watch than the eyes at first. Click when the patient moves his nose toward you, then toss a treat behind the dog so he turns away. Next, click for the dog looking at you, then approaching one step. Again, toss the treat behind the dog so he turns away. By tossing the treat behind, you're setting up the dog for a new repetition. By now, some patients will be running right up to you, while others will need you to reinforce each step toward you incrementally until they are ready to come all the way to you. Avoid reaching toward the patient while training approaches. First, we will teach the patient to come to you, then we will let him initiate touch through targeting.

Some patients will require an entire session just to train approaches, while others will approach within a few seconds. Be sure to note in the medical record what you did during the session, where the animal's skill level began, where it was when you concluded the session, and what your plan is for the next visit.

Video 7.1 shows a short shaping and targeting session with Fifi, a nine-year-old poodle with no history of training and moderate to severe stress in the veterinary clinic. This is her first time hearing a clicker, and her first training session. Each time she glances at or approaches Monique, she earns a click and a treat. In a few repetitions, she is too nervous to take the food, but she eventually approaches and even offers the target behavior.

Targeting

Once the patient will approach, we will invite them to a designated area using the foundation skill of targeting. When we say "targeting" in this section, we will refer to touching your hand, or a target stick or other object of your choice. For simplicity, each of these items will be interchangeably called a target.

Many of these patients have a learning history where the veterinary team member reaching for or touching them predicts something scary happening. Instead of reaching for the patient, let him come to you. For the first few repetitions, roll the treat behind the patient to send him away from you. Sending the patient away uses both food and increased personal space to reinforce the target behavior. If you need to move your hand or body, use the same treat-rolling process to move the patient away from you, then make your movement(s) while the patient is further away at first.

Using a similar procedure to training approaches, sit or stand near the station and hold your target (hand, stick, spoon, etc.) slightly away from your body. Watch for the dog to look at the target. Click, take the target away, and toss a treat. Remember: the click should happen during the desired behavior (the glance at the target), and the treat will come after. When the dog turns around, present the target again and click for movement toward the target. Each time, roll the treat past the dog to move him away and set him up for a new repetition. When he turns back toward you, present the target. Eventually, he will be ready to sniff or touch the target. When he sniffs or touches the target, click, remove the target, and drop a treat. The click should occur the *instant* his nose is touching the target. Once the dog has eaten the treat, present the target again, click for a nose touch, remove the target, and treat. By removing the target after each click, you are establishing that the target *appearing* is the cue for the behavior. You may also want to use a verbal cue in addition to the visual cue of the target appearing. A common choice is the word "touch" or "target." If you'd like to use a verbal cue, introduce it when the animal is starting to offer the target behavior frequently, and give the verbal cue at the same time you present the target.

After the dog has become comfortable touching the target, it is time to teach him to follow. If you're sitting, you may need to stand so you can move and he can follow. If you change body positions, reward a few simple targets in your new body position before trying to teach the dog to follow. Even something as simple as the trainer moving from a sit to a stand can change the dog's comfort level and emotional state. Present the target, and as the dog approaches, move the target 1" further away from him, to encourage him to move toward the target to touch it. The instant he touches the target, click, remove the target, and treat. Step by step, begin moving the target 2", then 3", then 4", reinforcing the behavior of moving to follow and touch the target several times at each increment. When the dog will follow the target for 5–10 steps, you're ready to use it to introduce the station.

Stationing

When deciding on what kind of station to use, such as a rug, mat, low platform, or table, consider what the end goal behavior will be. For a small-dog procedure, a cat procedure, or a medium-sized dog for cephalic venipuncture, an elevated platform may be helpful. For larger dogs, or procedures done from above such as eye and ear medicine or subcutaneous fluids and injections, the floor may be a better place to work. Choose a spot that will be comfortable for both the trainer/handler and the patient. Some patients may need to learn more than one station. For example, the table might be used for a physical exam, but the floor for a nail trim. Each time you change the station, you will need to retrain that behavior, so try to plan ahead and know in advance what you will want and need from the learner (refer to Figure 3.22 for station examples).

One approach to teaching stationing is to use the foundation target behavior to show the dog how to go to the station. To use a target to build stationing, first sit or stand near the station. Reward the dog several times for following the target, then move the target toward the station. When the dog places a paw on the station, click and treat. In this situation, treat the dog while he is in position on the station rather than tossing or dropping the treat behind the dog. Then have the dog follow the target to move off of the station, click, and treat in position. Move the target over the station, so the dog follows and places both front paws on the station. Click, and treat with the dog in position on the station. Move the target off of the station, click, and treat. Progress moving the target further and further, until the dog has all four feet on the station. Reward in position, and then reward again right away for remaining on the station. Repeat the process until you can reward every 3–5 seconds for remaining on the station to help build duration. Table 7.4 shows one example of a possible training plan worksheet for a session teaching stationing.

Video 7.2 shows using a target to move a Level Three dog to the station, and then introducing duration on the station by clicking and treating for the dog remaining on the station.

Stationing can also be trained using shaping rather than the target. Shaping to the station may be simple if the dog is already proficient in the shaping process, but will take longer if shaping is a new idea.

To use shaping, break down the behavior of "go to the station" into many building blocks, such as "look at the station," "move one step toward the station," "move several steps toward the station," "place one paw, then multiple paws, then all four paws on the station," and finally "remain on the station for longer and longer periods." When shaping, watch for the dog to constantly be trying to improve on the prior performances, and attempt to solve the puzzle. The dog should seem interested, engaged, and happy. If the dog checks out, seems uninterested, or begins offering the incorrect behavior, assess yourself and the process. The rate of reinforcement may be too low, which means you're expecting big steps instead of baby steps. The solution in this case is to split those steps into smaller approximations. The dog may not be offering improvements because he doesn't understand the shaping process, or that you're working toward a larger goal behavior. The dog may also be mentally fatigued, or stressed by the process. In that case, take a break, work on another behavior, check for environmental stressors, or stop the session.

Video 7.3 shows using the shaping to station exercise to teach Kyrie to move onto the table. Because the table is tall, an intermediate step of the bench is used to allow the dog to get all the way up to the table. This dog is going to learn to do voluntary cephalic venipuncture, so a table is chosen as her station, but she is uncomfortable with being lifted, so she is taught to go to the station on her own using shaping.

First the technician clicks and treats for looking at the bench, then for moving toward and touching the bench, then for touching the bench with a paw raised off the ground. The trainer raises the criterion here to paw behaviors only, ceasing to click for looking

Table 7.4 Sample of a possible Level Three training plan to introduce stationing.

Training plan: Level Three training	
Completed behavior: Go to station and remain there until end of behavior is signaled	Component behaviors: Look at station Move toward station Lean over station with any body part Any one paw Both front paws Any 3 paws All 4 paws All 4 paws, short duration All 4 paws, lengthening duration NO treat when off station
Consent point: All 4 paws on station	Consent point: N/A
Preferred reinforcers 1. Cheese 2. Bacon 3. Kibble	
Medications: None	Working area: Exam room 2
Foundation behaviors required: Clicker charged Hand target Approaches	Known cues needed: Sit, Hand target Additional DS/CC/CCC: Yes XX No
Starting criteria	Look at station
Progression	Patient progressed through all component behaviors as expected until duration was introduced.
Ending criteria	4 paws on station for 3 seconds
Observations	Patient relaxed and comfortable throughout the process, but showed mild loss of interest when duration increased beyond 3 seconds. Attempted to extend interest/working period using cued behavior of "sit" and "touch" when on station, but duration still not available.
Homework	Work on sit, touch, down, and building the repertoire of known cues so we have more alternatives for ping-pong and maintaining behavioral momentum.
Plan for next visit	Increase duration on station, introduce body touching on station if patient is comfortable.

or nose touching. The criterion is then raised to placing a paw on the bench, and then two paws. When the clicks stop for two paws, the dog rightly guesses to put all four paws on the bench. Once she will get onto the bench, the criterion is changed to moving toward the table. She then moves toward the table and touches it with her nose, her chin, and then a paw. The criterion changes again to paw touches only, and the reward is placed on the table to help promote correct guesses. The criterion is changed once again, this time to two paws on the table. Finally, the dog hops all the way onto the table, and earns a nice little jackpot of treats.

Training Tip: Two Strikes and You're Out

Maintaining a high rate of reinforcement and a low level of confusion is critical for training success, especially for new learners and new trainers. If an animal makes two errors in a row, pause, assess the situation, and split the criteria down into smaller pieces that are easier for the animal to understand. Multiple errors in a row will decrease behavioral momentum and slow the learning process.

7.6 Teaching Consent, Touch, and Restraint

Consent at the Station

Once the dog will go to the station, it is time to teach her she is in control of the interaction, and her way of controlling the interaction is by using the station behavior. The station becomes the on and off switch for interaction and rewards, and the animal will learn she is in charge of this switch fairly quickly. Video 7.4 shows a 16-week-old puppy being introduced to the station. She is reinforced when on the station with clicks and treats, but the clicks and treats stop when she is off the station. Even when lured with a treat, after only a few repetitions she clearly prefers to stay on the station.

When the patient goes to the station, click and treat for stationing, and then give a cue the animal knows well such as sit, down, or shake. Click and treat, repeating several times. Then use a target or tossed treat to move the dog off the station, and cease all clicking and treating. No reinforcement for being off the station. Move nearer the station yourself, and when the dog goes to the station, repeat the process of asking for several simple behaviors the dog knows well, and click/treat for each repetition. Generally during this process, the dog will choose to move off the station at some point. Perhaps she will be distracted by an odor, curious about something happening outside the room, or just looking for something else to do. When the dog opts out, leaving the station, it presents an opportunity to teach the dog no reinforcement is given for being off-station. Ignore the dog. Do not speak to her, pet her, or offer any treats or toys. If the dog leaves the station for more than 30 seconds, say her name and offer a target to move back onto the station. If she moves to the station, click and treat, and resume training. If she chooses not to return to the station, simply wait, give the animal a break, or end the session.

If the patient chooses to leave the station in the middle of training, pause and reflect on what just happened. Did you reach for the animal? Was there a noise outside the room like a barking dog? Did the owner move around or rattle the treat pouch? Have you been working for several minutes and the animal is mentally fatigued? Did the pet's paw slip or any other unsettling movement happen while she was on the station? Use what you learn to increase future success. If it was a reach toward the pet, we need more training on touch. If a dog barking outside was upsetting, remember to feed every time the patient hears that sound until she is no longer bothered by barking. Remember to make notes in the medical record for future sessions about what is successful, but also about anything that causes a pause or setback in training.

When the learner realizes he or she is in control of the training process by choosing to station, or choosing not to station, the need for distance-increasing signals and aggression falls away. We have established a new way to communicate, and the animal will learn we are listening to them. The animals can be excellent teachers for us, just as we can be for them, with mutual communication.

Stationing is only one kind of consent behavior, but it is the simplest one to teach, so we use it the most for examples in this book. Other consent behaviors include chin rest, holding on target, or changes in body position. We will introduce those concepts later in this chapter.

Teaching Touch

Once the patient will come to the station, and understands the interaction ends if they leave the station, we are ready to begin training to allow touching. For dogs, touching the front of the chest between the front legs is generally a good place to start, while cats usually prefer cheek or chin touching.

To begin teaching touch, invite the animal to the station. Watch the patient closely, and reach out to touch them. If the patient stays at the station and looks relaxed, touch in a nonthreatening way. Click *while* you are touching the patient, then treat. The click should mark the instant the touch is occurring, not the time after the touch has already stopped. In some cases, early in the process, the animal may move slightly when you reach to touch them. Click during every touch, and treat after every touch, even if the animal moves. As the patient becomes more familiar with the process, you will be able to increase criteria and click/treat only when the patient stands still for touch in the future.

If you reach out to touch the patient and they look nervous and lean away or start to move away, stop reaching toward them. This patient needs desensitization and classical counterconditioning to hand movements prior to touching. Move gradually through an exposure ladder for reaching and touching, with each step predicting a click and treat. Start by raising your hand an inch or two from your side, then click/treat. Continue moving your hand toward the patient a few inches at a time, until you can touch the patient. Remember: desensitization should look boring while it is happening. The patient should not show any signs of avoidance when you raise and move your hand. If the patient is showing avoidance or stress, make your hand movements smaller. If any hand movement at all causes stress, go back to asking for simple behaviors at the station, then end the session. Consider slowing the training plan and spending more time targeting where the patient touches you, modifying the environment to be less stressful, modifying the medical management portion of the treatment plan, or some combination of these suggestions.

Once the animal can tolerate reaching out, begin nonthreatening touches. Gradually lengthen the duration of the touch, and glide your hand over more parts of the body before clicking and treating. Begin touching in a less sensitive area, and glide to more sensitive areas, paying attention to any special concerns such as paws. For instance, if a patient has a strong fear response to nail trimming, wait to introduce paw touching until the patient is very tolerant of a full exam. When the animal has become comfortable with full-body touching, add a second hand to the touching process. Change between hands, and then touch with both hands. For some animals, touching with both hands is considerably different than touching with one hand. One hand means petting; two hands mean an exam or restraint. Train for this eventuality. When you're touching the patient with two hands, you may need to place the clicker under your foot, or change to a verbal marker such as a tongue cluck or the word "yes."

To keep pets interested, patient, and relaxed, play a little "ping-pong" when training touching behaviors. To play ping-pong, practice with touches, but between practicing touches, ask for other simple behaviors and tricks the patient knows. This builds **behavioral momentum**. Behavioral momentum is helpful because one success leads to another, and it encourages the patient to stay interested and engaged. By giving the learner some variety, we also reduce the pressure of learning to tolerate something scary (touches), and diffuse some stress before it builds. This process also normalizes touching into "just another trick," rather than having it seem suspicious or always predicting an exam or other potentially unpleasant experience.

Training for Sedation and Restraint

Some patients are so nervous that the most realistic behavior for us to train will be tolerance for sedation. In other cases, the patient may be able to learn voluntary treatments over a lengthy series of visits, but the owner may not be ready to pursue a long-term training relationship. For these patients, the most practical course is to teach cooperative sedation protocols.

For sedation, some dogs may first need to learn to wear a muzzle. See Section 7.7 for information on muzzle training.

The purpose of sedation training is to create a safe, low-stress experience for the patient, the veterinary team, and the client. Some animals can be trained to accept unrestrained sedation or walking sedation, while others are best trained for light restraint and then injection. When training restraint for injection, determine where the animal will be when sedated, what position the animal will be in, and how the handlers intend to touch the animal to sedate him. How many hands will you use to touch him? Where will your hands be? How many people will be present? How many people will touch him? Where will the injection be given? How long will the injection take? The answers to these questions will guide your plan for each specific patient's sedation training.

The least stressful position for restraint is generally standing or sitting for dogs, and sternal recumbency for cats. These positions are comfortable for the patient and give good access to the epaxial and gluteal muscles. Some sources recommend epaxial muscles as the preferred site for intramuscular injection, while others suggest gluteal muscles. In any case, it is important to make sure the patient is comfortable with the injection process to reduce patient movement and decrease the risk of potentially serious side effects from intramuscular injections. As with any protocol, pay attention to the animal's signals and be prepared to try something different during the training process. A few dogs may prefer to sit or lie down rather than stand.

> **Training Tip: Medication Makeovers**
>
> Training patients to accept sedation will result in patients who are less stressed and less fearful. Because these patients are more relaxed, they often require lower doses of sedation than they did when they were more fearful. Make sure to calculate drug dosages for the more relaxed patient in front of you rather than simply repeating what was done in the past when the patient's anxiety level may have been much higher.

For this example, we will discuss standing light restraint for a medium-sized dog for intramuscular injection.

Here are some example building blocks for this behavior:

- Come to station with syringe visible in training area
- Allow touching
  - Full body with one hand
  - Full body with two hands
- Allow touching under the neck and over the shoulder with one hand
- Allow touching under the abdomen or over the planned injection area with one hand
- Allow simultaneous touching of the neck and the abdomen
- Allow touching of the neck and abdomen with a light squeeze
- Allow squeezing of the neck and abdomen with gentle pressure
- Allow gentle-pressure squeezing for progressively longer durations
- Allow long-duration gentle pressure while a second person is in the room
- Allow duration pressure while a second person holds a syringe
- Allow duration pressure while a second person approaches with a syringe
- Allow duration pressure while a second person touches
  - Touches of injection area progress in firmness up to a pinch
- Allow duration pressure while a second person simulates injection with a capped needle
- Allow duration pressure during an injection.

Each of these steps is introduced gradually, and every small approximation is followed by a click during handling, and a treat afterward. If at any time the dog tries to move away or leave the station, he is allowed to do so. The temptation to keep going once we have our hands on the animal can be very strong. Remember how much effort we have invested to gain the trust of this animal. Trust comes with routine, predictability, and consistent mutual respect, and the desired behavior gets stronger through reinforcement of good approximations. Table 7.5 shows a sample worksheet for a training session to prepare a dog to allow sedation.

Video 6.6 showed Kylie accepting an intramuscular injection. She has been trained to respond to the cue "hug" to accept restraint. This is an example of a mixture of Level Two and Level Three training. Kiley gives consent for the injection behavior by pressing her body against Alicea, showing she is ready for the injection.

Video 7.5 depicts a very anxious and frightened dog named Charley. Charley suffers from many anxieties, and among them is fear of the veterinary hospital. Although he has been given pre-visit medications and had training visits with the technician, he is still very anxious, so the decision is made to train him for sedation rather than trying to continue with cooperative care training. His fear is simply too severe.

Table 7.5 Sample of a possible Level Three training plan for session 2 of 3 for IM sedation.

Training plan: Level Three training	

Completed behavior:
  Allow IM sedation
  Session 2
	Component behaviors (approximations):
	  Station – train in advance
	  Light body hug – train in advance
	  Touch injection area
	  Pinch injection area
	  Second person approaches with syringe
	  Second person pinches injection area
	  Faux injection with capped syringe
	  Actual injection

Consent point:
  At station
	Consent point:
	  Stands still without moving away

Preferred reinforcers 1. Peanut butter spoon 2. Squeeze cheese 3. Chicken baby food	
Medications: Trazodone night before and 2 hours prior	Working area: Exam room 1

Foundation behaviors required:
  Station
  Hug
	Known cues needed:
	  Sit, Hand target, Down, Spin
	  Additional DS/CC/CCC: XX Yes – 2nd person and all touching break down DS/CCC simultaneous with OC.

Starting criteria	Station and light hug, second person holding syringe
Progression	Patient progressed through approximations as expected, including faux injection
Ending criteria	Faux injection with capped syringe
Observations	Patient relaxed and comfortable. Second person approaching needed to be broken down so that we reinforced after each step she took toward the dog. Faux injection was well tolerated.
Homework	None required
Plan for next visit	IM sedation for exam, blood draw, radiographs

Alicea is the trainer in this video, and she starts by teaching hand targeting, and how to follow the target to the table. Charley is anxious, but chooses to participate rather than opting out of training. Once he remains on the table rather than immediately moving off, repeated hand targets are used to build duration, and then he is asked for some easy behaviors he knows like "sit."

When Alicea tries to bend over and pet him low on the chest, he shows avoidance behavior. She changes her plan, using a type of touch his owners say he is comfortable with. Using the same touch every time, the trainer clicks while she is touching, and then gives a treat. Charley looks stressed during the touch, but excited during the click. This is as close to a nonstressful starting point as this dog will get inside the hospital.

During the next session, the goal is to enter Charley's personal space, and touch him in novel ways. Charley targets Alicea's hand when she moves into his space, but when she touches his side, he refuses food, a sign of increasing stress. Changing tactics, the trainer uses hand targeting to build a trading-touches scenario: I touch you, you touch me, then click/treat. Once Charley is more comfortable, he can take treats for side touches again.

At the next session, Charley is taught to allow touch with two arms and the introduction of mild pressure. Although he is still anxious, he has the option to leave by moving off the station at any time, and he chooses to continue to participate. When he is tolerating the simulated restraint, a second person is added who will be giving the injection. The team works with Charley on approximations, building up to pinches over the injection area and simulated injections with a capped needle.

On the day of Charley's sedation, he is nervous but cooperative. He moves to the station, allows the hugging restraint, and lets the second technician approach. Charley does respond to the sting of the injection, but he rapidly returns to baseline and accepts treats again.

Note: This animal is receiving light sedation, and has been given several small treats. In the authors' combined experience (35+ years), this has never caused a problem. To minimize concerns about food ingestion and sedation, some practitioners prefer a liquid treat such as frozen broth, baby food, or licks of a thin canned food or gruel.

7.7 Muzzle Training

Consider this: a fearful, defensively aggressive dog is presented to the hospital. To stay safe, the team member grabs a muzzle and applies it with some difficulty. The dog is then held down by two people, while a third cleans his painful infected ear. The predictor of the stressful and painful experience is the muzzle. When the dog sees a muzzle in the future, it may trigger a strong response. Muzzle training can prevent these experiences.

Muzzle training is a good option for patients and trainers who feel better with a "safety belt" in place, to keep everyone safe if a mistake occurs. In some cases, when a muzzle is placed, everyone is more calm and relaxed around the dog, which can improve the dog's ability to relax as well. Muzzle training is an excellent idea for all dogs, not just anxious dogs. This training prepares them for possible times a muzzle might be required in the future. Teach owners to keep a properly sized basket muzzle in the pet first aid kit. If a pet sustains a painful injury, a muzzle can keep the owner safe during transportation and the veterinary team safe during assessment and pain management. However, the dog must allow placement of the muzzle for it to work.

Muzzle training is a variation on target training. Instead of targeting a hand, target stick, or spoon, the dog is taught to target the inside of the basket with his nose. Many dogs learn to love this game, and happily "get dressed" on cue. Creating this positive emotional response is far preferable to classically conditioning the negative emotional response that is so common.

To train application of the muzzle, use shaping and reward successive approximations. Place the muzzle on the floor or a chair, or hold it in your hand. During muzzle training, the goal will be for the dog to choose to put his nose into the basket, and never for you to reach toward the dog to push the muzzle onto the dog. Use the same process as teaching a hand target, but the goal is for the dog to go to the muzzle rather than the hand. Always use a basket-type muzzle, unless there is a strong existing unwanted emotional response to a basket. Basket muzzles allow the patient to breathe normally, pant, eat treats, and give social signals. Nylon quick muzzles do not carry these same benefits.

Here is an example of approximations leading up to voluntary muzzling:

- Look at the muzzle
- Look at and approach the muzzle one step, then two steps, and so on until he is close enough to touch it
- Touch any part of the muzzle with the nose
  - Begin clicking only for touches near the opening, then at the opening
- Place nose 1" inside basket, then 2", 3", and so on until all the way into the basket
- Place nose inside basket and allow basket to hang on nose for 1 seconds, 2 seconds, 3 seconds, and so on
- Allow basket to hang while strap is manipulated
- Allow strap to touch neck while basket is on nose
- Allow straps to meet behind neck while basket is on nose
  - Alternative: train closing the straps around the neck as a separate behavior, without the nose inside the basket, then combine both skills in later approximations
- Allow straps to meet behind neck while basket is on nose and buckle closed
- Gradually increase duration that the muzzle is in place

 Video 7.6 shows introduction of muzzling for a puppy. Teaching puppies to wear muzzles helps them see this is just one more normal part of life, and wearing something is no big deal; plus, it is a fun shaping exercise for the trainer and the puppy.

7.8 Physical Examination Training

There are many right answers when it comes to how to train a physical examination.

Some exams can be trained using the touching method described in Section 7.6, simply expanding the touches to include all aspects of the physical examination. Other patients might do best with individual cues for each portion of the exam, asking for presentation of specific body parts. Yet another set of patients may be most successful if taught a behavior like the chin rest or extended target for examination (see Section 7.11).

Touch Training for Exam

Physical examination is a series of touches. Using the principles of desensitization and counterconditioning introduced in Chapter 6 for Level Two exams combined with the Level Three touch-training protocol will often result in successful examination training. As always, the key is to progress at a pace that feels comfortable for the patient, maintaining a nonstressful experience, and where the goal behavior is broken down into its many building blocks, with each block representing an opportunity for reinforcement.

For physical examination using touch training, the consent point is staying at the station (or chin rest, target hold, etc.). Invite the animal to the station, and ask for a few well-known easy behaviors. When the dog is working well, begin practicing touch training as described in Section 7.6 to assess the patient's comfort with contact. When the pet seems comfortable based on food acceptance, body language, and staying at the station, initiate touches that are part of a physical examination.

As with the Level One and Level Two physical examinations, begin with less sensitive areas, progressing to more sensitive areas. Save any individual sensitivities, oral exam, paws, rectum, and painful areas for last.

During training sessions, the technician will both train the patient and observe responses, assessing for changes in the patient's stress level. Increases in the stress level are a sign to break down the touching into smaller increments, before the animal withdraws consent by leaving the station.

Begin touching in a less sensitive area, and then glide to the desired exam area. Gradually increase criteria for both pressure and duration as the patient becomes more comfortable. Timing is important: the click should occur at the end of the touch but while your hand is still in contact with the animal. Ping-pong between exam skills and other known behaviors such as "sit," "down," and tricks; this will help keep the session less stressful and more interesting. Also, giving the animal frequent breaks away from the station is important early in the training process, until their mental and emotional stamina is sufficient to work through an entire exam.

Training Tip: Maintain Your Momentum

Remember: known cues are secondary reinforcers. A patient who has learned to sit, touch, lie down, and go to mat has been given a primary reinforcer such as a treat for these behaviors many times. Often, being able to do simple behaviors in response to cues improves the animal's emotional state, and builds behavioral momentum. Keep your learner's momentum high by giving known cues intermittently during training sessions for new skills.

Here is a sample progression of criteria for the touch method exam training. Notice many of the steps have substeps built in. "Auscultation" as a step is too big. Split touches like auscultation into smaller approximations, then build up to the full diagnostic touch. If the animal appears to have an increase in stress, break down the behavior into even smaller approximations so the animal has a chance to learn the exam will be nonthreatening.

- Touch shoulder, glide to prescapular lymph nodes (LN)
- Glide to prescapular LN, palpate gently
  - Gradually increase pressure until diagnostic palpation is achieved
    - Do not increase continually; click and treat for every small pressure (criterion change)
- Move to submandibular LN, repeat process
- Touch hip, glide to popliteal LN
  - Gradually increase pressure until diagnostic palpation is achieved
    - Do not increase continually; click and treat for every small pressure (criterion change)

- Touch shoulder, glide along spine
  - Gradually increase pressure until diagnostic muscle and comfort assessment achieved
- Touch shoulder, glide to lateral chest where auscultation would occur
- Wear a stethoscope in your ears and repeat
- Hold stethoscope in your other hand, repeat
  - Approach with stethoscope
  - Place stethoscope next to the touching hand
  - Gradually increase pressure and duration until auscultation is diagnostic
  - Glide stethoscope to new locations for continued diagnostic auscultation
- Touch shoulder, glide down spine to flank, glide down flank to abdomen
  - Gradually increase pressure with one hand until diagnostic pressure achieved
  - Add a second hand at lower pressure
  - Gradually increase pressure of both hands until diagnostic pressure achieved
  - Do not increase continually; click and treat for every small pressure (criterion change).

Continue with each component of the examination, until every component has been trained. Some patients will be able to work through a full physical examination in one training visit. For others, the training process may require several visits before the technician can complete a full examination. Once the technician can perform the examination, it is time to involve the veterinarian and begin transferring these skills to a second person. Some patients will readily transfer these skills, while others will take more time to feel comfortable with a new person. Remember: we are making a long-term investment in the patient's welfare, allowing for a lifetime of faster and better veterinary care. For patients with individual sensitivities, for example those who are more anxious about the oral examination, it may be best for the technician trainer to display the oral cavity to the veterinarian, rather than having the veterinarian touch inside the patient's mouth.

Video 7.7 shows Coco, a very nervous Australian shepherd during two visits, one year apart. Coco trusts the technician due to their relationship based on positive experiences during handling training, but she is still frightened of the veterinarians.

In her first visit, Coco is still very nervous, so Alicea makes sure she holds all of the food, and uses the food to help keep Coco in a position where all veterinary team members will be safe if Coco goes over threshold.

In the second visit, one year later, the technician starts by warming up Coco for her exam, assuring she is ready to work and comfortable with coming to station and being touched, palpated, and examined. Coco shows mild stress markers, but chooses to stay on the training station and continues accepting food. When the veterinarian approaches, Coco stays at the station, but she shows her teeth and growls, signs of moderate and severe stress. The veterinarian is a savvy trainer. She pauses, approaching, and turns away while Alicea clicks and treats Coco for looking at the veterinarian, and then allowing her to approach.

The veterinarian can now approach, and begin offering treats. The physical exam is performed, and Coco earns clicks and treats for each phase of the examination. Notice the clicks happen *during* the touches. Coco is attentive to the veterinarian, and begins working for her as well as working for Alicea, which is a great step toward transitioning care. When it is time for Coco's vaccinations, Alicea administers them. Coco's established relationship with Alicea is more solid, and more likely to recover from a few sharp needles. Her relationship with the veterinarian is still new and a bit tenuous, so this was the better option.

Video 7.8 shows Penny, a mixed-breed dog who is in moderate to severe distress. She intermittently refuses treats, chooses to move away from the trainer, is crouched, trembles, avoids eye contact, leans away, and has a tucked tail, a tense face, and dilated pupils. She shows learned helplessness, which is a sign of severe distress. This video shows an examination that was needed due to an acute illness. Remember: patients like Penny may appear cooperative, but should be provided with anxiety-relieving medication and be prescribed interventional Level Three training to improve their veterinary care experience.

Video 7.9 shows Bija, a small mixed-breed dog with a history of defensive aggression and fearful behavior at the veterinary office. This video shows his progression through five visits, culminating with the veterinarian performing most of a physical exam. Monique is the technician trainer in this video.

During the early visits, a combination of desensitization and counterconditioning and operant conditioning are used. The technician breaks the examination process into its component parts, and introduces Bija to the desired responses during examination. At first, Monique works with Bija by performing the approximations as well as clicking and treating. Soon, the owner is brought into the picture. Monique and the owner communicate, so that the technician can do the exam, and the owner can click and treat.

During the final clip, Monique demonstrates to the doctor how Bija has progressed, and how he expects his examination to feel. As Monique demonstrates a portion of the exam, the owner clicks and treats, and the veterinarian replicates Monique's movements. Near the end of the examination, Bija becomes more nervous because the veterinarian moved a bit too quickly for his comfort. Even with this error, Bija was able to return to baseline and finish his visit.

In Video 7.10, Kismet, a Belgian malinois, has her first training visit for cooperative care. Kismet is familiar with training outside the hospital, but displays severe distress when she goes to the veterinary office. She was referred to us for cooperative care training prior to returning to her regular veterinarian. While she becomes still at times (this is common for the breed during touching), she chooses to opt in by coming to her mat and voluntarily participates in a simulated examination and injection preparation. Monique involves Kismet's owner in the process, so she can learn the techniques and apply them at home and with her regular veterinarian.

Naming the Examination

An alternative, or extension, of the touching method is the *named examination*. For the named exam, each portion of the exam is put on cue. The patient learns each cue predicts a certain part of the exam, and can be better prepared to participate (Figure 7.5).

To use this method, make sure you initiate touch in the same fashion each time you work with the animal. Say the name of the body part you're going to examine ("ear," "eye," "belly," "teeth," "heart," etc.) using the same sound and tone of voice each time you say it. Reach for the body part using the same movement and gesture consistently for each repetition. This is establishing both a verbal and a visual cue for the animal about what is happening next. The process will look like:

- Say "ear."
- Touch shoulder, glide to the ear.
- Click while ear is touched.
- Stop touching the ear, and give a treat.

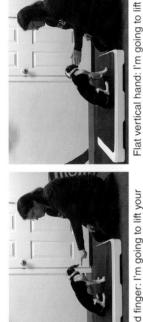

Hand over head: I'm going to touch your nose.

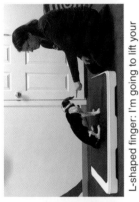

L-shaped finger: I'm going to lift your leg at elbow.

Flat vertical hand: I'm going to lift your ear.

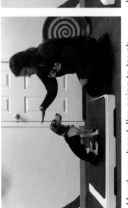

Pinching motion with fingers: I'm going to tent your skin.

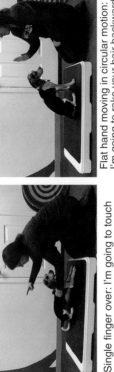

Single finger over: I'm going to touch injection site.

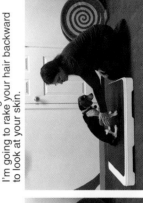

Flat hand moving in circular motion: I'm going to rake your hair backward to look at your skin.

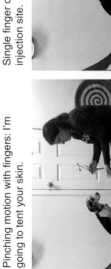

Presentation of stethoscope: I'm going to touch you with this.

Flat hand presented low: Give me your paw to touch.

Flat hand presented close to body: I'm going to palpate your belly.

Figure 7.5 Named examination example cues.

After a few repetitions, the animal will often begin pressing the cued body part toward the trainer, for example leaning the ear into your hand, leaning his chest against the stethoscope, or turning his rump closer to you for abdominal palpation.

Video 3.10 in Chapter 3 showed a demonstration of naming the physical examination with Millie. Notice the order of events is cue, touch, click while touching, reward.

For very sophisticated trainers, each portion of the exam can even be shaped into a separate behavior, or trick, of presenting the cued body part. For example, I would cue "teeth," and the dog would place his chin on my hand to offer an oral exam, rather than just allowing me to touch his teeth. I would cue "heart" while holding out my stethoscope, and the dog would press his chest to the stethoscope. Dogs can even be trained to open their mouths, and hold them open for a detailed oral examination (see links in the Appendix). The limit to what can be trained is only the physical ability of the dog and the sophistication of the trainer's skills. The process of presenting every body part is an extensive and exciting training project, and would warrant a whole separate guide of its own!

7.9 Treatments, Sample Collection, and Imaging

The recommendations for some treatments will sound familiar to you from Chapter 6, because desensitization and classical counterconditioning will automatically occur when we are using operant conditioning as well. Once the pet learns how to participate in his care and receives plenty of rewards for meeting criteria, he will be developing learned skills through operant conditioning, but also a positive conditioned emotional response, a sign of classical conditioning.

Subcutaneous Injections

Level Three subcutaneous injections build on the training we have done so far of stationing and touch training, combined with desensitizing the injection equipment and sensation.

Invite the animal to the station, and begin the familiar touching routine. Determine where on the body the injection will be given, and focus touching in that area, then begin expanding touches to tenting the skin. Remember: every approximation or building block earns a click and treat. When the skin tent is going well, introduce the syringe approaching, an injection with the capped needle, and finally the injection itself. Naming the injection procedure helps to establish a cue, so the pet knows what to expect during future sessions.

Once the injection procedure is trained, only a few clicks and treats will be required to perform the unrestrained injection.

The more savvy a patient becomes to training, the more quickly training will progress. During her examination training in Video 7.10, Kismet shows how quickly teaching a clicker-savvy dog's first exposure to subcutaneous injection training can go. This video also illustrates how quickly the animal can become comfortable when the environment is nonstressful and the patient has a good set of foundation behaviors.

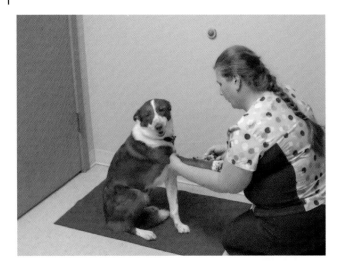

Figure 7.6 One example of a position for cooperative cephalic venipuncture training.

Cephalic Venipuncture

For cephalic venipuncture, the patient will need to be at a comfortable height for the technician to perform venipuncture. This may mean the floor or a table depending upon the size of the patient and the height of the technician (Figure 7.6). Foundation behaviors for cephalic venipuncture include stationing, paw target, and the touching exercise. Care should be taken, because we will be working face-to-face with unrestrained patients. Pay attention to food acceptance, body language, and proximity preference. If the patient looks uncomfortable or delays in participation, pause and assess the situation. Make sure to work safely while training.

The key to success will be breaking down the behavior into a series of building-block approximations, and then walking the patient through the approximations in a predictable way, clicking and treating for cooperation with each step.

Here is a sample of possible building blocks for the cephalic venipuncture behavior:

- Come to station
- Sit
- Present limb
  - First the paw, then the wrist, then the entire forelimb
- Rest limb on technician's arm
- Verbal cue and visual cue are introduced
- Allow technician to touch elbow
- Allow occluding vein while touching elbow
- Rest limb while vein occluded and palpated
- Rest limb while alcohol applied
- Rest limb during pinching of the skin and touching with capped syringe
- Rest limb during blood collection
- Rest limb during pressure application following blood collection.

 Video 7.11 shows training cephalic venipuncture for Rye. He is a clicker-savvy dog and learned the behavior from start to finish in two short sessions. This dog is generally cooperative for veterinary care and comfortable in the clinic, but is sensitive to needle

sticks. As Monique walks him through the steps, she uses his understanding of paw targeting, adding duration and building a complex behavior to show him how to cooperate for this procedure.

In the first clip, he is working on the table, and in the second clip he is working on the floor. The consent point for this dog is if he chooses to move to any position other than the sit. If he wishes for the process to stop, he can simply stand – he does not even need to leave the station for the procedure to stop.

Watch his body language. Notice he is mildly concerned about the procedure, but he is engaged in training and freely chooses to participate without any restraint. The second clip includes him giving his first unrestrained blood sample. He notices the needle stick and does not like the sensation, but remains stationary and cooperates, happy to accept his food reinforcement at the end of the behavior. Cooperative care may not make every patient love needles, but allowing them to have control over the process is what cooperative care is all about.

Video 7.12 shows Alicea working with Coco the Australian shepherd. Coco has completed her exam, and needs to give a small blood sample for a heartworm test. Coco already knows how to come to station and how to offer a paw from her prior nail trim training, and has a trusting relationship with Alicea for training in the hospital.

Coco is savvy to the veterinary care training process, and this session progresses quickly. Alicea is able to ask for Coco's paw, glide up to her elbow, hold off the vein, simulate a blood collection, and then collect blood. The consent point for this behavior is Coco offering her paw. She can withdraw consent by retracting her paw. In this video, alcohol is not applied. When using alcohol, incorporate it into the training process at the point you normally apply alcohol. Some technicians apply before palpation, and some after. Simply ensure the steps of training mirror your usual routine, so the process becomes familiar to the patient.

Video 7.13 shows Kyrie, a cattle dog, participating in cooperative cephalic venipuncture. Kyrie gives consent for this procedure by moving onto the exam table and presenting her front leg. Through progressive approximations, Alicea teaches Kyrie each step required to give the blood sample, culminating in Kyrie providing a fully cooperative sample.

Lateral Saphenous Venipuncture

For lateral saphenous venipuncture, at least two people will be needed: one to provide a target and observe the patient, and another to collect the blood. It is difficult to observe the patient's expression while working alone with a rear limb, but in calmer dogs it may be possible. Many dogs who are nervous will be reluctant to have us working around their hind limbs, and will prefer cephalic sampling. For a standing voluntary lateral saphenous, utilizing a hand target or chin rest can be very helpful. See Section 7.11 and the Appendix for more information.

Ear or Eye Medications

Ear and eye medications are similar to injections and venipuncture, an extension of the stationing and touch training. First, the patient will come to the station, then become accustomed to remaining at the station and holding still during eye or ear medications.

Training this skill is especially useful for patients who will be receiving chronic medications, such as those being treated for dry eye and KCS (Keratoconjunctivitis sicca), requiring lifelong daily eye drops.

Here is an example list of possible building blocks for the eye drop behavior:

- Come to station
- Touching of the head
- Gliding touch to the upper eyelid
- Raising the upper eyelid
- Touching the head while holding drops in the opposite hand
- Gliding touch to the upper eyelid and raising it while holding drops
- Applying a drop to a less sensitive area
- Applying a drop to the eye.

This list should look familiar; it is similar to the desensitization and counterconditioning list for this same treatment. The difference here is that if the animal moves away, no click and treat will occur. The patient is being given the opportunity to cooperate by coming to the station, giving consent, and holding still, rather than being taught to simply have a pleasant conditioned emotional response to receiving eye drops.

Video 7.14 shows a cat learning to accept ear medications. In the before video, you can see the staff is chasing Mama Kitty around the hospital to try to capture her and apply her ear medication. Mama Kitty is a clinic pet and very comfortable in the hospital, but still fearful of ear medications.

Alicea trains Mama Kitty using operant conditioning to follow her target, jump onto the table to station, and gradually allow the placement of medicated drops in the ear. While Mama Kitty moves away slightly during a few early repetitions, notice she is unrestrained and free to leave, and she can jump off the table to withdraw her consent to participate at any time. She chooses to stay engaged and an active participant in her own care.

Video 7.15 shows Rye; this time, he is learning to present for eye medications without restraint. Rye is savvy to veterinary training and to the clicker, but he has never received eye drops of any kind before this video. The video shows the power of good foundation behaviors, including the station and the understanding of veterinary training. Notice Monique tries to keep her cues consistent for the eye drop behavior, and the saline is dropped on less sensitive areas first before it is dropped into the eye. You will also notice the use of a verbal marker intermittently, when both of Monique's hands are needed for the procedure.

Imaging

Positioning for radiographs requiring lateral and dorsal recumbency can be stressful for any patient. Cooperative care training allows us to prepare animals in advance, so that in the event they require imaging such as this, they understand the environment and skills required. Remember: cooperative veterinary care can be prevention as well as intervention.

Video 7.16 shows an 18-week-old puppy learning cooperative positioning for radiographs. Before trying this on the x-ray table, Monique taught this puppy how to move onto her side when she said "night night," as a trick around the house and then on the floor of the veterinary hospital. This is her first session on the x-ray table. Kestrel gives consent to participate by placing her front feet on the table edge and allowing herself to be boosted onto the table. She is comfortable offering known behaviors like sit and down, so cooperative lateral recumbency is cued and reinforced. The V-tray is also introduced, but it is awkward for Kestrel to roll herself onto her back because of the shape of the tray. Monique gently helps her onto her back, and then using a combination of luring, targeting, and modeling, Kestrel is able to understand how to remain stationary on her back without restraint. As Kestrel becomes comfortable, duration is increased and the sound of the x-ray rotor is introduced.

Small variations in the environment can influence a learner's ability to understand cues and participate in training. In the second half of the x-ray positioning video, personal protective equipment such as a lead apron, thyroid shield, and lead gloves are introduced. Kestrel learns to understand the "night night" cue even when given with a gloved hand, and remains stationary while Monique puts on and takes off her gloves, simulating what will happen during a real x-ray. Finally, Kestrel earns clicks and treats for remaining in position while the trainer is in full PPE and the rotor is activated.

Emergency Sedation

In some situations, Level Three dogs may have medical needs that demand immediate treatment. These dogs will generally need sedation prior to treatment, and it is important to have an emergency sedation strategy for these rare events. Figure 7.7 shows positioning techniques for emergency sedation. Notice the dog is muzzled, he is wearing slip leashes, and he is being walked in a very distracting environment. A second team member is approaching him from the side, and will inject the sedation. In situations like this, taking the time to palpate the muscle prior to injection will often provoke an unwanted response from the patient. Simply inject as quickly as possible. Based on extensive experience, the authors have yet to see an adverse reaction with this technique.

(a)

(b)

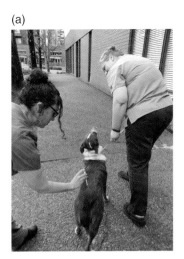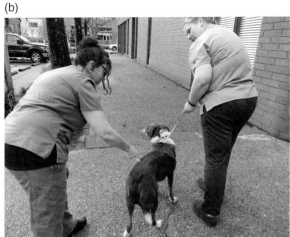

Figure 7.7 (a–b) Emergency sedation technique for dogs. *Source*: Courtesy of DeGeorge.

Author's note: Still images are provided rather than video for this procedure, because this scenario is so uncommon in the authors' respective hospitals. When we are presented with a Level Three dog who needs emergency sedation, the priority is always the welfare of the animal rather than capturing video, and adding a videographer to the situation may unnecessarily increase the dog's anxiety level.

7.10   Grooming

While we are not groomers by trade, veterinary professionals are equipped to provide these services for patients with special needs, such as Level Three dogs and cats. These patients need treatments like nail trims and anal gland expression, but are not good candidates for the untrained owner, or groomers not familiar with desensitization, counterconditioning, and operant conditioning techniques. Poor grooming experiences can cause considerable lasting emotional harm to patients, compromise the relationship between clients and pets, and damage the trust between veterinary professionals and patients. Teaching voluntary grooming behaviors improves the quality of care, and quality of life, for these patients.

Nail care is a prime topic to focus on for voluntary grooming. To trim nails, we will follow the same process used for other treatments. The behavior of nail trimming should be broken down into its small component building blocks, or approximations, and then the patient should be trained to participate in these approximations. If the patient chooses to opt out by moving away from the station, nail trimming should stop, even if the procedure has not been completed. Involving the owner in the training process will often create a functional situation where the owner can take over this routine care procedure at home, reducing the need for the patient to visit the veterinary hospital for nail care.

The example approximations for nail trimming are similar to the exposure ladder for desensitization, but the patient will need to agree to participate in each step to earn a click and a treat, rather than the steps simply predicting the appearance of food (Figure 7.8). Remember to give the patient frequent breaks, only progress at

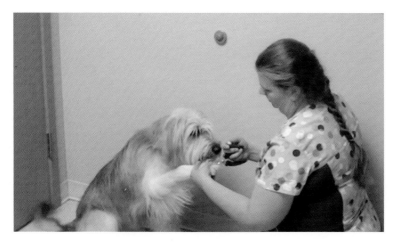

Figure 7.8 Example of cooperative nail care training.

the pace the patient is comfortable, and alternate or ping-pong with other behaviors during the training process to reduce stress and keep the training process fun. Table 7.6 shows a sample worksheet for a Level Three training session on nail trimming.

Table 7.6 Sample of a possible Level Three training plan for session 1 of nail trimming.

Training plan: Level Three training	

Completed behavior:
  Nail trim all 4 paws
  unrestrained
  Session 1
	Component behaviors (approximations):
	  Station
	  Offer or allow paw pickup
	    DS/CCC may be needed
	  Isolate toe, toenail
	    DS/CCC may be needed
	  Clippers to toe
	  Clippers around toenail
	  Sound of clippers near toenail
	  Tactile of clippers tapping nail
	  Clip one nail
	  Clip multiple nails
	  Repeat process for each limb

Consent point:
  At station
	Consent point:
	  Offers or allows paw handling

Preferred reinforcers 1. String cheese tiny bits 2. Chicken breast cubes 3. Cheerios	
Medications: Zylkene daily, Trazodone 2 hours prior	Working area: Exam room 3

Foundation behaviors required:
  Station
  Limb handling
	Known cues needed:
	  Sit, Paw target, Hand target
	  Additional DS/CC/CCC: XX Yes – Paw, toe, toenail may all be
	  needed

Starting criteria	Station
Progression	Station, shoulder, elbow, carpus, paw, toe, toenail, clipper approach
Ending criteria	Clipper tap on toenail
Observations	Pet was comfortable all the way until isolating a toenail. Toenail isolation was mixed with other skills – sit, hand target, paw target, and spin to decrease possible anxiety and preserve behavioral momentum. Mild stress (lip licks) at sight of nail clippers, but willingly targeted nail clippers with her nose. Ended by tapping toenail with clippers. No nail clipping performed today.
Homework	Owner OK to simulate training seen today, but do NOT clip any nails.
Plan for next visit	Clip one or two nails

Example building blocks for nail trimming:

- Patient comes to the station
- Touching begins in a less sensitive area, shoulder for forelimbs, hip for hind limbs
- Glide touch to the elbow or stifle
- Glide touch to the carpus or hock
- Glide touch to the paw
- Pick up nail trimmers in your other hand, and begin touching process again at the shoulder or hip
- Gradually progress to touching the paw
- Increase duration of paw holding
- Isolate a toe
- Isolate a toenail
- Increase duration of toenail hold
- Approach toenail with clippers
- Tap toenail with clippers
- Encircle toenail with clippers
- Trim one nail
- Trim multiple nails

Video 7.17 shows desensitization and operant counterconditioning for a canine nail trim. Douglas, the dog in the video, has bitten his owners when they try to restrain him for nail trims. He was calmer as a puppy, but as he grew and heavier restraint was used, he became more and more fearful for this procedure. You will see the technician provides a mat, which is the station area for Douglas. If he chooses to walk away and leave the mat, training stops, and when he returns, training resumes. The owners are present and observing as the technician works through an exposure ladder for trimming the nails.

Notice the dog's body language. A few mild stress signals, but he is overall nice and loose with a swishy wagging tail and eager for treats. After the technician demonstrates the technique, she then trains the owners to be able to simulate this technique at home. There is a considerable change to Douglas' body language when the owner attempts the training process. This is likely because the technician has never tried to trim his nails before, so there is no existing negative emotion associated with Monique touching his nails. There is significant unpleasant learning history from when the owner has tried in the past. Douglas still chooses to remain engaged and participate in training, staying on his station and cooperating. With the technician coaching, the owners work together, one handling and the other treating, accomplishing the goal of a nail trim. Pay attention to how nervous the female owner gets when she is told she can trim a nail, and then how happy she is when she successfully does so. Experiences like this improve the quality of life for patient and client, and help bond clients to the practice.

Video 7.18 shows a team attempting to find a comfortable procedure for puppy Chloe's nail trim. Multiple types of treats are offered, as well as working on the table, in a technician's arms, and on the floor. When she is on the floor, she begins accepting food, so this is the preferred location to work with her. This puppy seems more stressed by the restraint than the actual nail trimming, so teaching her to allow nail trimming without restraint is a key for success.

Fast forward six months, and the owner brings in Chloe for a nail trim, saying she "just could not trim the nails at home." Unfortunately, after the first successful nail trim, the client was not given enough information to perform cooperative nail trimming at home. She meant well, but had tried repeatedly to restrain Chloe and force her to accept nail care, causing significant aversion to the procedure. Chloe was signed up for training visits, and the second clip shows her participating in an unrestrained nail trim when she had a painful ingrown toenail.

Nail Boards

An alternative to conventional nail trimming is to teach dogs to file their own nails using a nail board. Dogs can be shaped to scratch on the rough board, filing their own nails using a scraping or digging motion. Figure 7.9 shows construction steps for making a nail board.

As with any shaping process, the completed behavior of scratching on the nail board is broken down into many component parts. These parts include approaching the nail board, touching it with any body part, touching with a paw, touching with multiple paws, moving the paw while touching the board, moving both paws while touching the board, and finally scratching at the board.

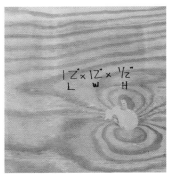

For strength use a 12 inch square of 1/4 inch plywood for the backer

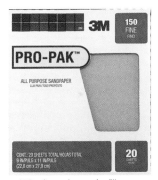

150 grit sandpaper for filing surface

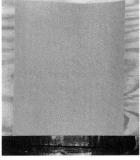

Tape sandpaper to plywood using duct tape

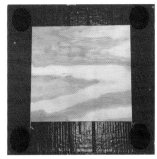

Rubber feet can be added to the back for traction

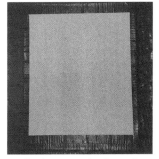

Sand paper can be changed as needed

Figure 7.9 Steps for constructing your own nail board.

Video 7.19 shows Alicea working through this process with a dog, using the principles of shaping to teach the dog how to file her own nails using the nail board. Notice how she gradually increases the criteria as the dog successfully understands each step, building a more complex behavior by starting with simpler ones.

Another alternative is to use a passive nail board. These boards are commercially available (brand name: BeckkyBoard) and are designed to be placed in a high-traffic area where the dogs frequently walk or run, such as a hallway or in front of a dog door. When the dog runs across the board, the nails are filed by the rough surface without any additional training required.

Other Grooming

Although grooming is not a veterinary procedure, Video 7.20 shows how to instruct clients to use desensitization and classical conditioning with a puppy for being brushed. It's a great example of stationing, shaping, desensitization, and counterconditioning.

7.11   Additional Consent Options

Stationing is a simple and easy way to establish consent, but it is only one of several commonly trained methods. One method that is based on zoo animal husbandry and is gaining popularity among trainers is called the chin rest. The chin rest is a behavior where the dog is in a standing or lying-down position, and is taught to target a towel, the trainer's hand, a pillow, the trainer's lap, or any other convenient surface with his chin (Figure 7.10). When the dog is keeping his chin on the chin rest, he is showing he is comfortable with the procedure and giving his consent. When he raises his chin from the chin rest position, he is communicating that he is withdrawing consent for that moment, and either the repetition was too challenging, more smaller steps are needed, his stress level has increased, or he is mentally fatigued.

Teaching the chin rest takes a little extra time compared to teaching a station, but it is an incredibly useful behavior because in the chin rest position, most procedures can be performed, including physical examination, eye medications, ear treatment and medication, vaccination, venipuncture, urinary catheters for male dogs, sedation, nail care, basic grooming, and other body-handling procedures such as fine needle aspirate, suture removal, hot spot treatment, and more. Any procedure that can be completed in the standing position and does not require access to the chin or ventral neck can be performed using the chin rest behavior with proper training.

The steps for teaching the chin rest include:

- Move toward the rest point
- Touch nose to the rest point
- Lean over the rest point
- Stretch neck over the rest point
- Touch chin to the rest point
- Maintain chin rest position for short durations
- Maintain chin rest point for extended durations
- Keep chin on the rest point while other procedures are introduced.

Figure 7.10 (a–b) Two examples of a chin rest behavior, one where the dog is standing and another where the dog is lying down.

(a)

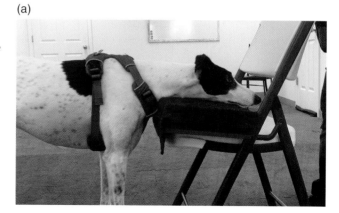

(b)

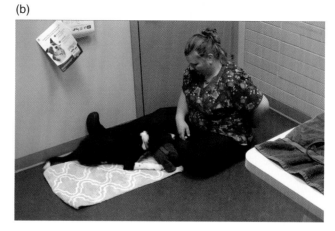

Procedures should be broken down into their component approximations, as discussed earlier in this chapter.

Video 7.21 shows Alicea working with her Greyhound to introduce the chin rest behavior. This dog's chin rest is placed on a chair, and shaping is used to help him understand how to move into the chin rest position, remain in the chin rest position, and control handling in the chin rest position by keeping his chin on the chin rest, or raising it to communicate he is uncomfortable with the treatment attempt.

Video 7.22 shows Monique introducing the chin rest behavior to her puppy Kestrel for the first time. The puppy is using a rolled towel as the chin rest for one session, and Monique's leg for a chin rest in the other session. This puppy is demonstrating the chin rest in the down position, an alternative to the standing chin rest. Choose a comfortable position for the patient that will allow the anticipated procedures in the future.

The Appendix contains links to videos by other trainers showing extensive training of the chin rest behavior.

Target Hold

Similar to the chin rest, the target hold is a consent behavior where the patient is asked to place his nose on a target such as the trainer's hand or a target stick, and remain in that position during treatment. If the patient removes his nose from the target, the procedure stops. If the patient keeps his nose on the target, the procedure continues. Refer to the Appendix for a link showing the target hold as a consent point for unrestrained anal gland expression.

7.12   Level Three Cats

As discussed earlier in this chapter, the veterinary environment presents unique training challenges due to the different social life of cats. It can be almost impossible to make the clinic environment comfortable enough for Level Three cats to engage in operant conditioning training. However, Level One kittens make excellent candidates to start with voluntary unrestrained care from the start.

One of the most useful skills to train for Level Three cats is voluntary carrier entry, and then planning for low-stress sedation strategies once the cat has arrived at the hospital. Shaping a cat to move into a carrier is simple, and can be done by almost any pet owner. Often, the best way to teach pet owners this process is by demonstrating with a comfortable cat, or providing video instructions. Video conferencing using internet or smartphone technology is also a great way to coach owners through training cats while allowing the cat to stay at home, where the stress level is low and the cat is comfortable.

Once the cat is shown to have no negative emotional response to the carrier (refer to desensitization and counterconditioning in Chapter 6), shaping to enter the carrier on cue may begin. For successful training, break the carrier entry behavior into many approximations.

Here is an example approximation list for carrier training (this also works great for crate training puppies and dogs):

- Cat looks at carrier
- Cat moves one step toward carrier
  - Cat progresses in one-step increments closer and closer to carrier
- Cat breaks the plane of the carrier entrance with his nose
- Cat places head in carrier
- Cat places head and one paw in carrier
- Cat places head and both front paws in carrier
- Cat steps with all four feet into carrier
- Cat moves far enough into carrier for the body, all four paws, and tail to be inside carrier
- Cat remains in carrier while door is closed

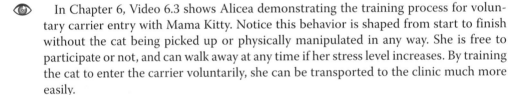

In Chapter 6, Video 6.3 shows Alicea demonstrating the training process for voluntary carrier entry with Mama Kitty. Notice this behavior is shaped from start to finish without the cat being picked up or physically manipulated in any way. She is free to participate or not, and can walk away at any time if her stress level increases. By training the cat to enter the carrier voluntarily, she can be transported to the clinic much more easily.

Level Three Cats with Medical Needs

In some cases, Level Three cats will present with true medical needs that cannot be postponed to allow training. In these instances, it is important to have strategies for how to handle the cats without worsening their anxiety whenever possible. Use all the principles introduced in earlier chapters to set up the environment to be as low-stress as possible, assure all your equipment is set up prior to handling the cat, and make a handling plan that allows minimal restraint and short procedures. Figure 7.11 shows one positioning technique for cephalic venipuncture in Level Three cats who prefer to hide.

Video 7.23 shows a cephalic blood draw on a severely stressed cat. This procedure was a need and not a want, as the cat is ill. Notice the cat is allowed to rest in the bottom half of his carrier and the blanket provides a pseudo hiding spot. The first technician uses her hand and the towel to gently rub the chin and be ready to provide restraint if needed while extending the front leg from the towel. Although the cat vocalizes some, he is cooperative, and the blood draw is performed with minimal additional stress.

Video 7.24 shows a subcutaneous injection on a severely stressed cat. Notice Alicea moves calmly but quickly to get the cat under a towel and ready for the veterinarian. As soon as the injection is complete, the restraint is over and the cat is free to leave.

Emergency Sedation Planning

Once a Level Three cat has been provided with pre-visit medications and taught to enter the carrier, she can be brought to the hospital and sedated as necessary for treatment. Refer to Chapter 3 for owner instructions on low-stress transportation practices.

Sedation should be rapid and quiet, using minimal contact and restraint. All equipment and medications required should be gathered prior to the patient's arrival, and a quiet room reserved in advance. Once the cat has arrived, the method of sedation depends upon the type of carrier used and the personality of the cat.

Figure 7.11 Positioning a cat under a towel for cephalic venipuncture. The towel protects the handler and the cat, and only the limb is exposed for blood collection.

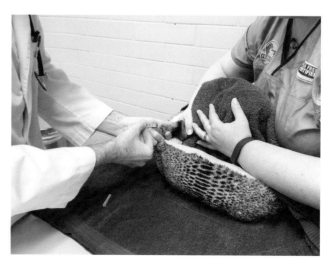

For soft-sided carriers, the cat can be sedated without leaving the carrier by injecting through the carrier's mesh (Figure 7.12). One team member will apply a thick soft towel or small blanket over the carrier and the cat, stabilizing the cat for the injection. A second team member can approach and rapidly administer an intramuscular sedative. Communication between the team members is crucial for this procedure to go smoothly.

For hard-sided carriers, the carrier can be disassembled, and a thick soft towel or small blanket used to sandwich the cat against the bottom of the carrier, stabilizing the cat to allow intramuscular injection (Figure 7.13). With this method, one team member

(a)

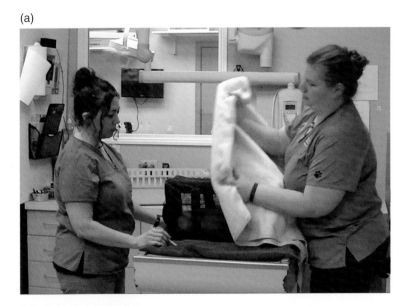

(b)

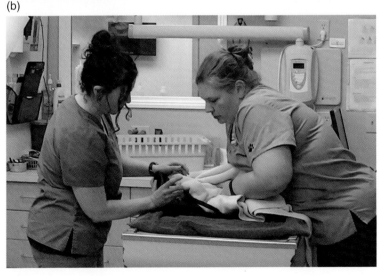

Figure 7.12 (a–b) Placing a towel over a soft-sided cat carrier and then administering emergency sedation.

(a)

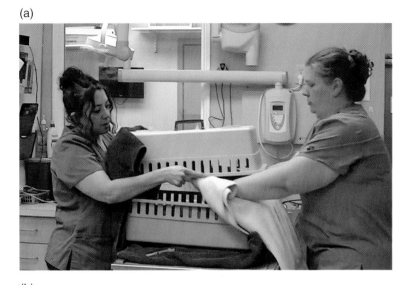

(b)

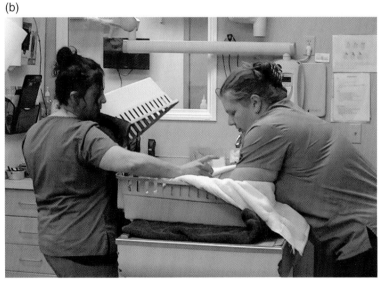

Figure 7.13 (a–b) Sliding a towel into a hard-sided cat carrier and then administering emergency sedation.

controls the lid of the carrier, while the second team member rapidly introduces the towel at the same moment the carrier is gradually opened. When the cat is stable, the team member who was controlling the carrier top then gives the injection. The carrier top is then replaced so the cat can fall asleep without further restraint.

Video 7.25 shows two team members rehearsing emergency sedation for a cat, first in a soft-sided carrier, then in a hard-sided carrier. This rehearsal is done using a decoy so the team members can practice their technique without causing undue stress to a live patient. Notice the towel used is large enough to cover the carrier and the cat, and thick

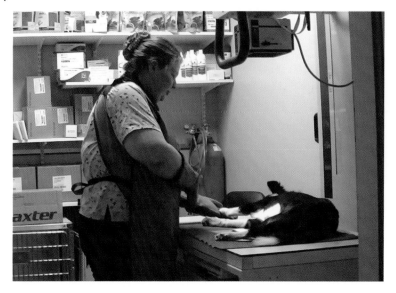

Figure 7.14 Voluntary lateral radiograph position training with a puppy as preventive care.

enough that even if the cat were to bite, no teeth could penetrate the towel. Once the first team member stabilizes the cat, she tells the second team member she is ready, and the injection can be given.

Part 2 of the video shows two team members practicing the sedation technique using a towel sandwich in the hard carrier. A decoy cat is used in this video for training purposes. Observe the team members working together to coordinate their timing, working quickly to minimize stress on the patient, and communicating quietly but succinctly throughout the procedure.

Conclusion

Level Three training isn't just for Level Three patients: every patient is a great candidate for fully voluntary care (Figure 7.14). However, Level Three patients require this type of interventional training because Level One and Level Two training efforts will fail due to their individual preferences, learning history, or both. Using operant conditioning combined with the principles of desensitization and counterconditioning is a powerful technique that empowers pets, facilitates cooperative low-stress and stress-free care, improves the quality of patient care, and helps clients feel more comfortable bringing pets to the clinic. Veterinary technicians, veterinarians, trainers, and owners can all learn to apply these cooperative veterinary care techniques to improve the well-being of animals.

8

Additional Patient Resources

8.1   Introduction

Training is an amazing tool to improve a patient's ability to cooperate for care and tolerate necessary treatments. In a perfect situation, every patient will respond well to training,
every client will support the training process, and every treatment can be completed
with zero patient stress. Rather than holding out for perfect, we need to be practical.
Some patients will require more than training in order to recover from prior stress or
trauma. Some patients will have fear responses that are so strong, it is impossible to find
a non-stressful starting point for training. Some clients will not have a desire to follow
through with training visits beyond training for sedation. Some animals are only semi-
domesticated, such as feral cats, and training is not an option.

   If you find yourself feeling stuck, as though you're not sure how to help a patient, or
how to best proceed, first remember to ***stop***. Do no harm. Consider what additional
services within the clinic and beyond may help this patient.

8.2   Neutraceuticals and Pharmaceuticals

The most common adjunct to training is medical management of fear, stress, and anxiety.
Medications should always be prescribed by a veterinarian, based on their assessment of
the patient. There are a wide variety of medications commonly used for animals, but few
FDA-approved medications for these indications in pets. However, widespread use has
shown these medications to be safe and effective in most cases.

   There are two basic medical modalities of behavioral medication in veterinary
medicine: baseline medications and event-based medications. There are also a variety
of supplements available for event-based or baseline use.

Baseline Medications

Baseline medications are prescribed by the veterinarian when patients require daily treatment for anxiety-related behaviors or disorders. Baseline medications fall into several
categories, but the most common category used in veterinary practice is selective serotonin reuptake inhibitors (SSRIs). Tricyclic antidepressants (TCAs), monoaminoxidase

Cooperative Veterinary Care, First Edition. Alicea Howell and Monique Feyrecilde.
© 2018 John Wiley & Sons, Inc. Published 2018 by John Wiley & Sons, Inc.
Companion website: www.wiley.com/go/howell/cooperative

inhibitors (MAOIs), and combination drugs are also selectively used in pets.[1,2] Because pets can't talk and tell us precisely how they feel during treatment, we must observe behaviors and infer whether the medications are helping the pet. The owner's observations are generally the most helpful, and the veterinary team can guide the owner's observation skills by teaching them what to watch for.

At the time of publishing, there are two baseline behavioral medications approved for use in pets: Reconcile® (fluoxetine, Elanco, suspended production) and Clomicalm® (clomipramine, Novartis). Both are approved solely for the treatment of separation anxiety.[3] For this reason, it is important to obtain consent from your clients for extra-label use of behavioral medications. There is one event-based medication approved for use in dogs: Sileo® (dexmedetomidine oromucosal gel, Zoetis). Sileo is approved for the short-term relief of signs associated with noise phobia in dogs.[4]

Many animals who are fearful in the veterinary hospital and anxious about treatment have concurrent anxiety in other contexts. Animals with global phobia, social anxiety disorders, separation distress, separation anxiety, social conflict, conflict aggression, fear-related aggression, cognitive dysfunction, noise phobia, and many other diagnoses are often prescribed a baseline medication.[1,2] A majority of baseline medications require 4–6 weeks to achieve stable serum levels and allow assessment for effectiveness. Most of these medications are established to have a wide margin of safety in animals and have published doses in most drug references (e.g., Plumb's[3]).

Pets who are prescribed a baseline medication *must* also be prescribed a behavioral therapy plan. The purpose of medication is to mitigate anxiety and fear to the point at which behavioral therapy is useful. Some animals require lifelong treatment, but others can be weaned off medication if behavioral therapy is sufficiently helpful.

Event-Based Medications

Event-based medications are short-acting anxiolytics that are used to briefly ameliorate predictable periods of anxiety. Most anxiolytics widely used in pets are in the family of benzodiazepines. Examples include alprazolam, clonazepam, lorazepam, chlorazepate, and so on.[1,2] Another event-based medication that is rapidly gaining popularity in veterinary medicine is trazodone, which is a tetracyclic antidepressant and SARI (serotonin antagonist and reuptake inhibitor).[6] The analgesic and anticonvulsant medication gabapentin is also known to affect GABA, and can reduce anxiety.[5] Beta-blockers such as propranolol and clonidine are also used as event-based medications in special circumstances.[7,8]

Training Tip: There Is No Magic Pill

Behavioral modification is the most important part of every treatment plan. Remember, the purpose of medications is to relieve suffering, improve welfare, and facilitate behavioral modification. There is no medication that will treat and resolve behavioral concerns without the benefit of a behavior modification plan.

Event-based medications can be given to pets who will be experiencing a sudden stressor. Examples include veterinary visits, travel, fireworks or other loud noises, unavoidable separations from dogs with separation distress, and exposure to any fear-provoking stimuli.

These medications begin working right away, and do not require administration for days or weeks to see a result. For veterinary phobias, administration the night before the appointment and again 2 hours prior to leaving home has been documented as a preferred protocol for many commonly prescribed anxiolytics.

Like any medicine, behavior medications will sometimes cause an unwanted reaction, or not be effective at the initial prescribed dose. For this reason, any event-based medication should be given as a test dose during a nonstressful period to assess for any unwanted response and see if the medication is likely to be helpful for the patient.

Often, pets with anxiety disorders are treated using both a baseline medication and an event-based medication for breakthrough stress. This is not usually indicated when anxiety is limited to veterinary phobias, but rather for disorders affecting the quality of the animal's home life. For example, a pet with separation anxiety is likely to take fluoxetine every day, but may require trazodone or a benzodiazepine for periods of unavoidable separation, especially early in the course of treatment.

Neutraceuticals

Neutraceutical supplements can also be helpful for veterinary phobias and other anxieties. There are many commercially available supplements for anxiety reduction. Some of these products have considerable effects with respect to serotonin and other neurotransmitters. Neutraceuticals should always be selected with the veterinarian's guidance. Many neutraceuticals are classified as dietary supplements, but they do affect neurotransmitters and can have synergistic effects with other medications as well as serious side effects. Always question clients carefully about possible over-the-counter product use prior to prescribing any supplements or medications to avoid drug or drug–supplement interactions. The most frequently discussed serious adverse reaction to behavior medications is called *serotonin syndrome*.[1] This syndrome can cause serious and even life-threatening clinical signs, but it is rare. Serotonin syndrome is usually a result of high doses of medication, or combinations of two or more serotonin-affecting medications or supplements (remember: medications such as mirtazapine, dextromethorphan, and tramadol are not behavior medications, but certainly affect serotonin).[1,3] It is important for veterinarian prescribers and veterinary technicians to understand the mode of action and what to expect when medications are prescribed. Proper client education is a key to appropriate therapy and avoiding serious side effects.

Acepromazine: Don't ACE Fear!

Acepromazine is a tranquilizer, but it does not treat anxiety.[1] Because acepromazine slows the body down but does not calm the mind, it should not be used as a single agent for the treatment of anxious pets. Imagine you're having a root canal. Because you move around too much, the dentist gives you some gas to make you feel a little groggy and then injects Novocain® to numb the tooth. Unfortunately, the injection doesn't work well, and you're in a lot of pain during the root canal. Because you're sleepy from the gas, you can't move and talk to object to the pain; you're too groggy to move much and show how upset you are. To the dentist, you look just fine, but you're becoming more and more fearful. Now, think about the next time you need to visit the dentist, even for a cleaning. You'll probably be afraid. The same thing happens when we give acepromazine to pets. They become groggy and slow in their movements, but their mental suffering is unchanged or, based on some studies, may even be intensified.[9]

8.3   Professionals and Their Roles

Every patient benefits when a full team of support is available. This team may include a veterinarian, a **veterinary technician**, a **veterinary technician specialist in behavior** (VTS Behavior), a trainer, a veterinary behaviorist, and/or an applied animal behaviorist. It is important for veterinary team members to understand the unique role that each of these professionals fulfills in caring for fearful and phobic patients.

The veterinarian's role is to diagnose conditions and prescribe treatment. If an animal has a behavioral disorder, such as separation distress, global anxiety, noise phobia, social phobia, and so on, this diagnosis should be made by a veterinarian. The veterinarian may be a general practitioner, a veterinarian who is also an applied animal behaviorist, or a veterinary behaviorist. Veterinary behaviorists are board-certified specialists in behavior. These highly trained professionals have completed a residency, and passed the rigorous examination to become diplomates of the American College of Veterinary Behaviorists. Veterinary behaviorists can provide additional support for any patients the general practitioner would like to refer.

The technician's role is to support the veterinarian and the client. For behavior patients, the technician will take a history, assist with examination, and educate the owner about the diagnosis, any medications prescribed, and direct implementation of the treatment plan. The technician can design treatment plans for patients requiring preventive care, but a veterinarian's orders are needed for patients requiring intervention. Veterinary technician specialists in behavior have completed extensive additional education in behavior, have a minimum of 4000 hours of clinical experience in behavior, and have passed the national board exam to be certified as members of the Academy of Veterinary Behavior Technicians. These highly qualified professionals may support the veterinarian with even the most challenging behavior patients.

A trainer or applied animal behaviorist can assist the owner with behavior modification and training, but should not diagnose behavioral disorders, nor recommend or prescribe specific medications. If a trainer or behaviorist is working with a client's animal and thinks the owner should explore medications, the client should be referred to his veterinarian for this service and discussion.

To assure every patient receives the highest level of care available, veterinary teams should take time to assure on-staff technicians are trained to educate clients about treatment plans, provide prescribed training, and educate clients about medications. Veterinary teams should be familiar with local positive reinforcement trainers, certified applied animal behaviorists, and veterinary behaviorists, so that an entire team can work together when necessary for patients who need collaborative care.

In some cases, the roles of technician, technician specialist, trainer, and applied animal behaviorist may intersect, just as the roles of veterinarian and applied animal behaviorist may intersect. It is important to remember the technician can provide a huge range of services for clients and patients, but must refrain from diagnosing disorders and prescribing medications. Refer to Table 8.1 for a summary of the qualifications for different behavior and training professionals.

Table 8.1 Breakdown of professionals recommended by the authors and their qualifications.

Behavior professional	Credentials	Degree required	Training school	Exam written/practical	CE	Code of ethics
American College of Veterinary Behaviorists	DACVB	DVM with residency	No	Yes/no	Yes	Yes
Certified Applied Animal Behaviorist	CAAB	PhD	No	Yes/no	Yes	Yes
	ACAAB	MS		Yes/no	Yes	
Academy of Veterinary Behavior Technicians	VTS (Behavior)	Credentialed technician	No	Yes/yes	Yes	Yes
Karen Pryor Academy	KPA CTP	None	Yes	Yes/yes	Yes	Yes
Certification Council for Professional Dog Trainers	CPDT-KA	None	No	Yes/no	Yes	Yes
Certification Council for Professional Dog Trainers	CPDT-KSA	None	No	Yes/yes	Yes	Yes

References

1 Overall, K. (2013) *Manual of Clinical Behavioral Medicine for Dogs and Cats.* St. Louis, MO: Mosby.
2 Shaw, K., and Martin, D. (2015) *Canine and Feline Behavior for Veterinary Technicians and Nurses.* Ames, IA: John Wiley & Sons.
3 Plumb, D.C. (2015). *Plumbs Veterinary Drug Handbook.* Stockholm, WI: PharmaVet.
4 Korpivaara, M., *et al.* (2017) Dexmedetomidine oromucosal gel for noise-associated acute anxiety and fear in dogs: A randomised, double-blind, placebo-controlled clinical study. *Veterinary Record.* 17 February, 7 pp. doi:10.1136/vr.104045
5 DePorter, T., *et al.* (2015) Tools of the trade: Psychopharmacology and nutrition. In *Feline Behavioral Health and Welfare.* St. Louis, MO: Elsevier.
6 Gruen, M. (2008) Use of trazodone as an adjunctive agent in the treatment of canine anxiety disorders: 56 cases (1995–2007). *Journal of the American Veterinary Medical Association.* 233 (12), 1902–1907. https://doi.org/10.2460/javma.233.12.1902
7 Ogata, N. (2011) The use of clonidine in the treatment of fear-based behavior problems in dogs: An open trial. *Journal of Veterinary Behavior: Clinical Applications and Research.* 6 (2), 130–137. https://doi.org/10.1016/j.jveb.2010.10.004
8 Overall, K. (1997) Pharmacologic treatments for behavior problems. *Veterinary Clinics of North America: Small Animal Practice.* 27 (3), 637–665. https://doi.org/10.1016/S0195-5616(97)50058-1
9 Endersby, S. (2014) Noise phobias and fireworks. *Veterinary Nursing Journal.* 29 (10), 332–334. doi:10.1111/vnj.12183

9

Implementation Strategies

9.1   Change Is Never Easy

Change is never easy. The uncertainty of change brings discomfort, fear, and anxiety for us, just like the veterinary setting can bring anxiety for some of our patients. Changing the entire veterinary industry's view of our daily patient interactions will take time, but the change has already begun. The authors feel privileged to be on the forefront of this change, providing education for veterinary professionals around the world with great pleasure. We have watched as the veterinary community has started to embrace the approach of treating the patient's mind *and* body. The desire to change for the better becomes stronger with each passing year, but perceived obstacles can slow or stall change if we are unprepared for them.

The single most important factor influencing successful change is clinic culture. The veterinarians and support staff must commit to making every patient experience as pleasant as possible, and to helping clients understand how deeply each of us cares for the total well-being of our patients. As the clinic culture begins to change, the team will start to feel the effects: fewer bites and scratches, fewer distressed patient vocalizations, fewer distressed clients, and improved satisfaction with how we interact with patients.

Next, clients will begin to notice. The client may make remarks like "Wow, he didn't even growl at you. He always tries to bite at the vet's office," or "I've never seen him so calm at the doctor's office." These happy clients will have happy pets who take up less time and effort for treatments. Happy clients will tell their friends about the great experience their pets have at your hospital, bringing even more clients who are interested in the very best care to your doorstep.

When the team and the clients all expect cooperative, low-stress care and positive experiences in the veterinary clinic, it is easy to provide this care. Unrealistic and outdated expectations are a primary obstacle to change. When the client comes to expect patient-centered low- and no-restraint care, we are obligated to be able to provide it.

9.2   Proposing Change

Achieving change "from the bottom up" can be a challenge. Most of our readers are probably veterinary support staff. As technicians, the authors understand how challenging it can feel to get managers and veterinarians to embrace change. Don't be

Cooperative Veterinary Care, First Edition. Alicea Howell and Monique Feyrecilde.
© 2018 John Wiley & Sons, Inc. Published 2018 by John Wiley & Sons, Inc.
Companion website: www.wiley.com/go/howell/cooperative

afraid to be the voice of change in your hospital. Advocate for your patients! Advocate for your patients in a way managers and veterinarians will embrace rather than resist: with a great plan.

Identify Solutions

The first step to change is identifying solutions rather than seeking out problems. A solution-based approach will promote cooperation and teamwork. A problem-based approach will often encourage defensiveness and resistance. No one likes to be told they are doing things wrong. One example of identifying a solution would be a proposal for nonslip surfaces. A problem-based approach would be to say, "We are supposed to have nonslip surfaces in the exam rooms and we don't, so the animals are struggling during visits." A solution-based approach would be "I have an idea to improve patient comfort in exam rooms, and it is simple: provide nonslip surfaces for them." While this may seem like a matter of semantics, *how* we say something is often more important than *what* we say when it comes to gaining support for change.

Start Small

Once you have moved through your practice and looked for the solutions you'd like to suggest, consider the impact each proposed solution would have on the practice, and rank them from lowest impact to greatest. In general, smaller changes are easier to make than larger ones. Trying to make a huge change will often meet with resistance, and then only be maintained for a short time before the clinic reverts back to the old way of doing things. By selecting small changes, it is easier for the team to adapt.

Breaking down change into small steps takes advantage of what we know about learning and shaping. Throughout this book, we have discussed desensitization and shaping. Both of these methods work because they take a larger stimulus or more complex behavior, and break it down into nonthreatening and achievable building blocks. The same technique works with veterinary teams. Break changes into smaller chunks to build larger change over time. For example, if the change we want to make is "Every patient has a pleasant visit every time," that change is too vague and too large to accomplish all at once. Instead, break it down into smaller ideas, such as improving exam room surfaces, providing a variety of treats in every room, or scheduling frightened cats at the end of the day.

In addition to the change feeling like a small task, some managers and veterinarians will appreciate less costly changes first, before making what feels like a large financial investment in something new. Veterinarians are well-known for being thrifty! When you are ready to propose a solution, make sure you calculate the anticipated cost of the change and present it with your proposal. When possible, projecting the anticipated revenue (if it can be quantified) will also help managers and veterinarians feel more comfortable.

Choose Measurable Changes

When embarking on the project of spearheading change, choose measurable changes at first. "Every patient, every time," is difficult to measure, because it is subjective and broad. At first, choose changes that will be easy to measure, and devise a system for measuring the effects of the change in advance.

If we continue with our example of nonslip surfaces, we can begin to build our proposal. You may go to your supervisor and propose adding nonslip mats to two exam

Table 9.1 Sample proposal worksheet: A worksheet to guide proposals for changes to promote patient-centered veterinary care at the hospital level.

Patient-centered care proposal		
Proposed change		
Incremental changes (if any)		
Date	Proposed start date	Assessment date
Assessment type	Assessment team	
Enhancements to patient care		
Enhancements to hospital, team satisfaction and safety, etc.		
Financial benefits	Financial costs	
Anticipated challenges	Marketing tools (if any)	

rooms for one month. You have already calculated how many mats will be needed and how much they will cost. How will you measure the effects of this change? By democratic vote. In the proposal, designate a time period, such as two weeks or one month, for the testing period for this change. In addition, designate a method to measure the change. In our example, we would suggest trying the mats for two weeks, and proposing a voting date where each member of the team is allowed to vote yes or no for keeping the change, and offer feedback if they would like to do so.

By making a formal and carefully thought-out proposal to leadership, you show you are serious about advocating for change. Your effort to include the entire team in the decision-making process will improve confidence and support, and will contribute to a positive change in clinic culture. Being organized, thoughtful, and inclusive are all good ways to gain support from management and make effective change over time. Table 9.1 is a worksheet for planning a proposal for change in your own practice.

9.3 Overcoming Obstacles: Common Concerns and Questions

As the authors work to spearhead change within the veterinary community, the same questions and perceived obstacles present themselves repeatedly. Be prepared to answer these questions for yourself and your team when you propose changes within your hospital. Recognizing these obstacles in advance will better prepare you and your practice for the changes ahead.

Perception: It's Too Costly

The costs of not providing patient-centered care will far outstrip the costs of doing so. Fees for equipment, treats, and team training are a small price to pay for increased client base, increased client satisfaction, improved safety, and improved job satisfaction.

To start, there is the cost of lost clients. How many clients do not return to the clinic after a negative experience? According to the Bayer/AAFP study, 58% of cat owners are reluctant to visit the veterinary office due to patient stress.[1] Losing clients due to perceived patient stress is a reality. Changing client perceptions of stress will encourage those clients to return to the hospital.

Providing compassionate and cooperative care requires fewer team members for a procedure. The ear cleaning and treatment that may have required three or four team members now requires only one or two. Working within the patient's comfort means low or no restraint. Manpower requirements are reduced by at least *half*. Reducing the number of team members required per procedure saves time and money.

Paying close attention to animal communication and working to keep animals comfortable and cooperative will reduce team injuries. Defensive aggression toward team members is a primary cause of injuries within the clinic. Injuries are costly for the hospital due to medical costs, labor and industry claims, and lost revenue due to employee absences.

Client loyalty and satisfaction are also increased when we work with the owner present. Clients understand more clearly the treatments provided, adding to their perceived value of services. When clients better understand and appreciate the treatments provided, we answer fewer financial concerns and complaints, saving the team time, money, and frustration.

While there is always some monetary investment with change, the money saved and improvement to the practice will make this one worthwhile investment.

Perception: It Takes Too Long

Using compassionate, cooperative, and low-stress methods really does not take more time. In the cost example, we discussed how fewer team members are required per pet when the pet is cooperative and calm. Returning to the example of a large dog with otitis, say three people are involved in restraint and one person is treating the ears, with the procedure taking 15 minutes. Multiplying 4 people x 15 minutes each = 60 minutes of team time. Consider also the time invested to figure out that four people would be required. Starting and stopping the procedure, relocating the patient to the treatment room, and pulling other team members away from other patients all cost time. If only two team members are involved, even if the procedure requires 20 minutes to allow for training, 2 people × 20 minutes each = 40 total minutes invested. Table 9.2 shows an example of the possible time investment and financial cost comparison associated with manual restraint and chemical restraint for a large dog's ear flush.

Using these methods also improves patient cooperation over time, decreasing the number of team members and time required for future visits. Investing some time and patience during our early relationship with patients sets us up for a future of efficient care, because animals are willing participants rather than defending themselves against us.

Video 9.1 gives an example of time comparison between the use of force and the use of cooperative methods for weighing a large dog. The first clip shows a team member lifting the large dog onto the scale. The second clip shows the second team member using her body in the correct position and a treat trail to lure the dog onto the scale in less than half the time.

Table 9.2 Risks, benefits, and associated costs with sedation for otitis treatment.

Procedure	Staff time required	Risks	Financial profile
Otitis treatment: conscious, active patient	20 minutes ×3 team members =60 total minutes	Patient injury Team member injury Iatrogenic behavioral injury Incomplete treatment Client perceives patient stress Decreased client trust	Team time cost = $20 Fee to client = $75 Profit = $55
Otitis treatment: sedated patient	15 minutes ×1.5 team members =22.5 total minutes	Adverse drug reaction (rare)	Team time cost = $7.50 Cost of medication = $1–10 Fees to client: Sedation = $50–120 Ear flush = $75 Profit = $117–177

This table uses an assumed hourly wage of $17 plus benefits for cost calculations.

Video 9.2 shows a completed trained scale behavior in an 18-week-old puppy. This puppy happily rushes in the door of the veterinary hospital to be weighed. Her training program incorporated classical conditioning and operant conditioning. Notice her positive emotional response in addition to her cooperative skill of moving onto the scale mat and lying down. Imagine a world where each of your canine patients makes weighing this easy!

Video 9.3 uses the example of removing a fearful cat from the carrier for an examina- tion. In the first clip, the technician tries to remove the cat through the door. First she coaxes, then she reaches, then she tries to dump the cat out through the door. Eventually she gives up, and the cat is still in the carrier. The second clip shows the same technician, same cat, and same carrier. In this version, she disassembles the carrier around the cat. This version requires less than half the time, and results in the technician being able to work with the cat.

Perception: But This Is How We've Always Done It

Veterinary professionals love animals. Our mission is to relieve animal suffering and improve animal well-being. Agreeing to change how we practice forces us to admit we have room for improvement. The emotions associated with this change, especially for established practitioners, can be complex. We may feel guilt for things we have done in the past. The screaming cats we have stretched, the struggling dogs we have forced into lateral recumbency while two people lay on them for grooming, the defensively aggressive dogs we have caught on a rabies pole or squeezed in a cage door while they urinated and defecated in terror, the cats we caught in an induction chamber and watched struggle and crash against the sides while they are induced – we each did those things because we had been taught it was for the best. We were told receiving veterinary care was in the animal's best interest in that time, no matter what was required to accomplish the goal. We may even have felt pride in being able to handle the most dangerous patients without being injured. It takes time to process these feelings of guilt and fear of change, and to embrace the idea of treating patients with a different mindset and aiming for a different result.

Criticism of people and their techniques will only worsen the guilt and fear into defensiveness and resistance. Successful change is built on recognizing strengths and positive actions, and building them up. Look for positive remarks to make. Some examples of positive remarks might include:

"I noticed you recorded in the chart Oscar did well standing while eating peanut butter for his blood draw. Thank you so much; we read it before we drew his blood today, and it made his visit go much more smoothly."

"Fluffy was showing really anxious body language when I walked by. It was great how you stopped trying to get the blood sample and Dr. Smith prescribed anxiety relievers."

"You have such a nice way of calming cats. Can you help me by feeding Precious while I try to give her vaccinations?"

If you know a certain team member is nervous around defensive dogs, or anxious around frightened cats, discuss these fears in a positive way. Acknowledge your appreciation for how sensitive the team member is to the patient's signals and body language, and reassure them they will not be required to participate in that patient's care until they feel relaxed and ready. Forcing team members to interact with patients they fear can predispose the team member to mistakes, and worsen anxiety for both pets and people over time.

Some team members may express concern about giving so many treats and so much food during visits. They may worry about gastrointestinal (GI) upset or nutritional imbalances. There are a variety of ways to approach this concern. First, your hospital can implement follow-up calls. Simply call and check on the patient the following day, and see if any GI upset or other side effects were noted. Lastly, you can cite the experience of experts. The authors have both conducted next-day calls to check for any trouble related to treats in patients, and have found rare instances of GI upset. Subjectively, these occurrences seem less frequent than stress-induced colitis or motion sickness was in the past.

Perception: I'm Not Sure What to Do

It is difficult to embrace change when we feel uncertain, and anything new always comes with some uncertainty. Providing standard operating procedures and a written standard of care, including a behavioral standard, will help clear up expectations. New team members should be provided with good training sessions, such as shadowing an experienced team member, and with excellent reference materials (such as this text!). Continuing education can be provided in-clinic, or by visiting conferences and symposia to help keep the team motivated and all on the same page.

Knowledge is power, and developing a united set of protocols for when to progress, when to stop, why to stop, and how to talk with clients will help decrease uncertainty and increase confidence and progress.

Lastly, you don't always have to know exactly what to do. You just need to know what is normal, what is abnormal, what is within your scope to treat, and where to refer cases when necessary. The team should be familiar with the nearest veterinary behaviorist who is a Diplomate of the American College of Veterinary Behaviorists. Furthermore, the team should be familiar with local applied animal behaviorists and local trainers.

If you don't have a trainer in-clinic for classes and skills, it is important to know how to choose a trainer for referrals. Trainers should embrace low-stress and positive reinforcement methods. They should be familiar with the principles of desensitization, classical counterconditioning, operant conditioning, and basic problem solving for pets. The trainer should have an open-door policy for observers, always welcoming clinic staff to come and watch, or potential clients to watch a class before signing up.

Perception: We Might Make Clients Angry

Veterinary medicine is a customer service industry. We have long been taught that the veterinarian knows best when it comes to diagnostics, surgery, and prescriptions, but in all other ways the client is always right. Furthermore, there is a long-standing dogma in the profession that we should be able to "do anything" to animals, because we "have a way with them." We must keep our eye on the most important aspect of the care we provide: being the best possible advocate for the animal.

Communication is everything when we are talking with clients about quality of care. The client may arrive with a goal-oriented mindset with a dog we haven't seen in two years. The client would like to have an exam, vaccinations, a heartworm test, fecal sample, vaccinations, a nail trim, and anal gland expression, and have the infected ears diagnosed and treated. A visit like this is unlikely to be completed all in one try, even for the most comfortable and patient dog.

The technician is the first line of communication in setting a good client expectation for this visit. Use a script such as "Dr. Jones is going to start with Fido's checkup. Based on what she sees, she will explain to you which treatments she thinks we should perform today when we start treatment for his ears, and which treatments would be better to do when we see him for his ear follow-up in 10 days." This script begins to introduce the client to the ideas of: wants versus needs, prioritizing care based on the animal's medical needs, and dividing care into more manageable segments.

During the examination, the veterinarian can continue this important message. "Mrs. Smith, I am so glad you brought Fido to see me. His ears are quite painful, and you're right, they are infected. Because his ears are painful, I'd like your permission to give him a pain reliever that will also make him feel sleepy. We can clean and medicate his ears, and collect his heartworm test and perform his grooming if he is staying nice and relaxed. When you return in 10–14 days, I'd like to give Fido's vaccinations after the infection has healed."

Additionally, the whole team can have a good script for if we need to stop. Be honest with clients. Express your empathy for the patient, pointing out signs of stress and fear to the client. Explain your desire to provide the very best care, which includes awareness of emotional harm we could be causing. Describe the importance of maintaining a good trusting relationship between the patient and the medical care team, so you can continue to provide a whole lifetime of excellent care for your patient. Showing clients that we care about patients, and we want to care about them for an entire lifetime, demonstrates how much we value both physical and emotional wellness in the hospital.

Finally, the team needs to be prepared to provide relief from stress and fear in the clinic, using short-term aids such as anxiolytic medications and long-term aids like training visits and happy visits, to achieve the goal of long-term stress-free patient care.

Perception: It's Hard to Know When to Say "Stop"

Knowing when to say "Stop" relies on every team member understanding the hospital's behavioral standard of care, and feeling empowered to prevent iatrogenic behavioral injuries (IBIs). Every veterinarian and every team member needs to be on the same page, and provide a united message with good continuity for clients. If one technician forcibly restrains a vocalizing puppy for vaccination, but the next technician refuses, both the client and the patient will trust us less. The client may say things like "He was fine last time," or "Just hold him down and do it quickly." These remarks are signs of a lack of continuity of message within the team rather than signs of a problem with low-stress techniques.

If this situation happens, always have a supportive message about your teammates. It can be easy to criticize a teammate without thinking about it. Even saying something as simple as "Jennifer is still learning" or "Maybe I can figure out a different way to do this" can damage the client's confidence in the team and sound judgmental. Focus on the animal in front of you, and remark only on what you can observe today as well as the proposed plan for today's visit.

Using the resources provided, propose adopting a behavioral standard of care for your clinic, focused on improving the patient experience, increasing team safety, and preventing IBIs. Figure 5.1 suggested a scoring system for the emotional state of pets, based on the levels of training we have introduced. This scoring system dovetails with the detailed flowchart provided by Dr. Colleen Koch we introduced in Chapter 4 (Figure 4.2). Use these to guide your decisions when filling in Table 9.3, a guide to making your own standard of care.

Perception: I Am Afraid …

Of being injured while working with an unrestrained animal.
Of being called a follower or part of a new "fad."
Of clients thinking I am afraid of patients.
Clients won't understand.

Table 9.3 Developing a behavioral standard of care.

Designing a behavioral standard of care

---

1) Review the hospital's mission statement; assure emotional wellness is included.
2) Select an assessment tool for measuring patient stress.
3) Determine "stopping scores" within your assessment tool (e.g., "Moderate" = pause).
4) Define exactly who can stop a procedure (everyone who handles patients).
5) Educate the team about the behavioral standard of care.
6) Educate clients about the behavioral standard of care.
7) Designate a person(s) to monitor patient care, and assure it meets the standard of care.

Use these steps to begin your hospital's journey toward adopting a behavioral standard of care for every patient, every visit.

Fear inhibits behavior in pets and people alike. Fear of working with unrestrained animals comes largely from being expected to get everything done during a single visit all the time, and without sedation or medications of any kind. Restraint beyond light stabilization is only necessary when animals are fearful and trying to escape or defend themselves. By carefully observing our patients, and training them, medicating them, and choosing not to push them over their threshold, we can remain safe while working with unrestrained animals. In fact, for both authors, each of the times we have sustained bites from patients, the patient was being heavily restrained and something went wrong. As of publication, neither of us have been bitten by an unrestrained patient, in over 35 years of combined experience.

Some clients may be judgmental if you change your style of care. The client may say that you're just trying to take part in a new fad, or you're afraid of their patient and can't handle him. In the 1890s, Ivan Pavlov began characterizing classical conditioning. *The Behavior of Organisms* by B.F. Skinner was released in 1938. Learning theory is nothing new. Taking the time to learn it is a new, widespread feature of veterinary medicine.

Our reluctance to push an animal over its threshold and force defensive aggression may read as fear or reluctance to owners, because they are accustomed to that type of care. Reiterate to yourself and to the client the purpose of stopping and making a new plan: to provide the very best care while causing the least possible amount of stress, improving patient wellness, and preserving the trusting relationship between veterinary professionals and patients.

Use direct education and passive education to teach owners what to expect at the veterinary hospital. Hang posters of relaxed and fearful animal body language cues. Provide handouts describing the special approach and services you provide. Create Purr Packs and Wag Bags that include: pheromone wipes, a neutraceutical stress reliever, a dose of anxiolytic medication, and instructions for a stress-free ride to the clinic. Post displays with flyers advertising your Purr Packs and Wag Bags in each exam room to start the discussion about comfortable care. If you need to reschedule a visit, communicate in advance with the client about any financial changes associated with additional visits so there are no surprises.

9.4 Making Change for the Right Reasons

Clients and team members will embrace the change to cooperative and low-stress care, and making prevention of IBIs a priority, when we approach it from a position of empathy and positivity. Every client who brings a patient to the hospital loves that pet enough to go to the trouble of coming in. If the animal is acting fearful or defensive, the owner may be anxious, embarrassed, or angry. Education is the key.

Demonstrate and teach empathy for these animals and their owners. Avoid labels like "bad," "mean," "tough," "spoiled," or "dominant." Simply describe what you see: an animal who stops taking treats, moves away, looks away, or becomes tense as a form of communication (Table 9.4). Translate for the animal, and communicate the meaning of these subtle signals to the owner. You're an expert! Show the owner each sign and signal, and explain that the patient is simply worried about what will happen next.

Table 9.4 Flipping the script.

Label	Example replacement
Bad	None (not an appropriate term for pets)
Dominant	None (not an appropriate term for pets)
Mean	Fearful, anxious, stressed
Fractious, aggressive	Fearful, anxious, stressed
Stupid	Incomplete training
Spoiled	Fearful, anxious, stressed
Stubborn	None (not an appropriate term for pets)

Avoid the use of labels for animals in the veterinary hospital. Instead, describe emotions or behaviors. Some terms have no replacement, because they are inappropriate for pets and especially for the veterinary setting.

Reassure the owner that you and your team are perfectly equipped with the tools and knowledge needed to help this patient, and you'll guide them through every step of the process together, even if it means more than one visit.

Conclusion

Our hope is this book has empowered you to look at your patients in a new light, and commit to giving every patient the best possible veterinary experience every time they visit the hospital. By improving awareness of patient sensation, perception, and communication; creating a behavioral standard of care; understanding learning theory; and learning about the training options and methods available, you're already off to an amazing start. We hope you are excited to work with patients who are less stressed, more relaxed, and willing to participate in their own care. We hope you are inspired to consider the more advanced training methods of operant conditioning and fully voluntary patient care for the future. And, lastly, we hope we have reignited your love of animals and reminded you of our true mission as veterinary professionals: to improve *all* aspects of the lives of animals.

Reference

1 Volk, J., *et al.* (2011) Executive summary of the Bayer veterinary care usage study. *Journal of the American Veterinary Medical Association.* 238 (10), 1275–1282. https://doi.org/10.2460/javma.238.10.1275

Appendix

Helpful Links and References

Veterinary Technician Specialists in Behavior

Academy of Veterinary Behavior Technicians
http://www.avbt.net

Continuing Education

Clinical Animal Behavior Conference
http://www.animalbehaviorconference.com

Fear Free Certification
http://www.fearfreepets.com

Additional Training Resources

Karen Pryor Academy
http://www.clickertraining.com
http://www.karenpryoracademy.com

READY ... SET ... FOR GROOMER & VET: HUSBANDRY TRAINING
Animal Behavior Training Concepts taught by Laura Monaco Torelli
http://www.abtconcepts.com/training-videos/

Pharmacology and Neutraceutical Resources

These are only a few examples. Behavior-specific texts tend to have the most relevant indications for use and dosage information.

Fear Free Certification: Library and Toolbox
http://www.fearfreepets.com

Cooperative Veterinary Care, First Edition. Alicea Howell and Monique Feyrecilde.
© 2018 John Wiley & Sons, Inc. Published 2018 by John Wiley & Sons, Inc.
Companion website: www.wiley.com/go/howell/cooperative

Landsberg, G., *et al. Behavior Problems of the Dog and Cat,* 3rd ed. (2013).

Overall, K. *Manual of Clinical Behavioral Medicine for Dogs and Cats* (2013).

Veterinary Information Network (Behavior Library and Behavior Boards) http://www.vin.com

Glossary

A

adrenaline As a response to stress, it is a hormone secreted by the adrenal gland that increases the blood flow, breathing, and metabolism to prepare the body for muscle exertion.

aggression Behavior intended to harm, or at least threaten to harm, another.

alpha roll An outdated practice of rolling a dog onto his side and holding him down until he submits. Research has shown this method can provoke aggression.

amygdala A small mass of gray matter inside each cerebral hemisphere associated with experiencing emotions.

anal glands Small glands found on both sides of the anus between the external and internal sphincter muscles.

analgesia The inability to feel pain. An *analgesic* is a drug that takes away pain or decreases it.

antecedent Anything that happens before the target behavior, such as a cue or a trigger. Antecedents can be environmental, gesture, sound, smell, person, and so on.

anxiety The feeling of nervousness, uneasiness, and apprehension often marked by physical signs.

anxiolytic Anything used to reduce anxiety, such as drugs, nutraceuticals, pheromones, and aromatherapy.

appeasement Behavior that an animal performs in order to decrease a threat from another organism.

approximation A step toward the desired behavior.

auscultation Listening to the heart and lungs with a stethoscope as part of the physical exam.

aversive Anything an animal deems physically or emotionally uncomfortable.

B

behavior The way in which an animal acts in response to a particular stimulus.

behavior modification The alteration of behavioral patterns through the use of learning techniques such as operant conditioning or classical conditioning.

behavioral momentum During training, asking for an easier behavior the animal already knows to increase reinforcement while working on more difficult behaviors.

Cooperative Veterinary Care, First Edition. Alicea Howell and Monique Feyrecilde.
© 2018 John Wiley & Sons, Inc. Published 2018 by John Wiley & Sons, Inc.
Companion website: www.wiley.com/go/howell/cooperative

binocular vision Where both eyes overlap, creating a field of vision with good depth perception.

body language Nonverbal communication, both conscious and unconscious.

C

calming signals See *appeasement.*

capturing Reinforcing an already known behavior to put it on cue. For example, waiting for a new puppy to sit and then clicking and treating the sit.

carpus Small group of bones comprising the wrist.

cephalic Pertaining to the head. The cephalic vein is a superficial vein that runs the length of the arm.

classical conditioning (also known as *Pavlovian* or *respondent conditioning*) The pairing of a neutral stimulus with an unconditioned stimulus; through repeated pairing, the neutral stimulus becomes a conditioned stimulus and elicits a conditioned response.

classical counterconditioning Changing the emotional or physiological response of an animal.

clicker A plastic and metal device that, once pressed, makes a clicking sound. After conditioning, it becomes a conditioned reinforcer.

cochlea The auditory portion of the inner ear.

compassion fatigue Compassion fatigue is best defined as physical and mental exhaustion and emotional withdrawal by those who care for the sick, dying, or traumatized. This disorder is prevalent in veterinarians, veterinary technicians, veterinary team members, shelter workers, and human healthcare providers.

conditioned reinforcer (also called a *secondary reinforcer*) A reinforcer that has acquired its reinforcing properties by being a predictor of a primary or innate reinforcer. Examples are a clicker, whistle, or other bridging stimulus.

conditioned response This is the response to a conditioned stimulus after classical conditioning has taken place. It is also the response of an organism after learning has occurred.

conditioned stimulus This is the stimulus that creates the conditioned response after classical conditioning has taken place.

cones A light-sensing cell in the retina of the eye, responsible for sharpness of vision and color perception in bright light.

confirmation The externally visible features of a dog or cat that appear to meet breed standards.

conflict Mental struggle due to opposing needs, such as when an animal wants to perform for treats but also wants to retreat from a fearful stimulus.

consent Giving permission for something to happen. In animal training, it is a behavior that has been taught to allow the trainer to touch or perform a procedure on the animal.

consequences Anything that happens immediately after the target behavior. The process by which these consequences influence behavior is called *operant conditioning.*

contingency A future behavior or circumstance that cannot be predicted with certainty. Also a provision for an unforeseen event, such as having a contingency plan in place for training.

cooperative care The animal either gives consent by performing a behavior or is easily distracted by food during veterinary procedures.

cortisol Hormone secreted by the adrenal gland in response to stress or low blood-glucose concentrations.

criteria Standards by which something may be judged or decided.

cue A signal that will elicit a specific behavior or reflex after learning has taken place.

D

defensive aggression Aggressive behavior motivated by self-defense in response to a perceived threat.

depth perception The ability to see the world around you in three dimensions and determine the distance you are to an object or another organism.

desensitization The decrease of an emotional response to a stimulus after gradual exposure.

differential reinforcement of an alternative (DRA) Reinforcing any behavior other than the target behavior you are suppressing.

differential reinforcement of an incompatible behavior (DRI) Reinforcing a behavior that is incompatible with the target behavior that you are working to suppress. For example, reinforcing sitting instead of jumping, because both behaviors cannot occur at the same time.

dilated pupils The widening of the pupils in response to the sympathetic nervous system being activated, medications placed in the eye, or lower light.

discriminatory stimulus A stimulus that signals that a behavior, if performed, will be reinforced or will not be reinforced.

displacement A behavior that seems out of context. For example, a nervous dog that play bows at a team member most likely is not trying to initiate play.

distraction techniques Using high value reinforcement to divert the animal's attention away from the procedure being performed.

dorsal Pertaining to the back of the animal. Dorsal recumbency is when the animal is held lying on his back.

dysphoria A state of unease, restlessness, depression, and anxiety.

dystocia The condition of having difficulty giving birth.

E

exposure ladder A hierarchy of feared stimuli used to systematically desensitize an animal to a feared stimulus; also known as a *parenthetical exposure hierarchy*.

extinction When behavior that was previously reinforced is no longer reinforced, it fades away.

extrinsic Not naturally occurring; this behavior would be taught and maintained by external reinforcement.

F

fear Emotional state caused by the belief that someone or something is a threat to the animal's safety.

fear period Developmental stages during which animals seem more susceptible to fearful stimuli, and a higher risk of a lasting conditioned emotional response from a short interaction exists.

fight-or-flight response An acute stress response originating in the hypothalamus in response to a perceived harmful attack or threat to survival.

flank The side of an animal between the ribs and hips.

flooding Exposure therapy where the animal is exposed full force to a feared stimulus until he stops reacting. This technique is considered inhumane and not used in veterinary medicine.

freeze response Sometimes added to the *fight or flight response*. When responding to a perceived threat, an animal may fight, flee, or freeze.

frequency The number of cycles per second (Hertz) of sound waves; the lower the number, the deeper the sound.

functional assessment An approach to figuring out why an animal performs a specific behavior, using the antecedent, behavior, and consequence model.

G

gastric dilation volvulus (GDV) Also known as *bloat* or *gastric torsion*. A life-threatening condition where the stomach twists and fills with gas.

genetic Traits that come from the lineage of the animal; also known as *hereditary*.

H

habituation After repeated exposure to a stimulus, the animal stops noticing due to the lack of reinforcement or punishment.

happy visit When a patient visits the veterinary hospital for the sole purpose of being reinforced with food, praise, and/or play, and leaves without having a procedure performed.

hock Sharp angled joint that is the ankle in dogs and cats.

home base In animal training, this refers to keeping your treat delivery hand in a neutral location before the click, so as not to distract the animal.

human–animal bond A mutually beneficial and dynamic relationship between people and animals that is influenced by behaviors that are essential to the health and well-being of both.

hypervigilance Exaggerated behaviors whose purpose is to detect threats. In dogs, these behaviors are usually pacing and scanning with eyes and ears.

hypothalamus Located in the forebrain, the hypothalamus controls body temperature, thirst, hunger, and other homeostatic systems, and is involved in sleep and emotional activity.

I

iatrogenic behavior injury A physical or emotional injury received due to fear, stress, or anxiety during a veterinary exam or treatment.

inhibited bite A bite that does not leave a mark on the skin of the receiver. Also called a *soft mouth* or *bite inhibition*.

intrinsic Naturally occurring.

J

jackpot When a leap in the training plan occurs or the goal behavior is performed by the animal, a trainer delivers multiple treats.

jugular vein Large veins of the neck carrying blood from the head toward the heart.

L

lateral Pertaining to the side of an animal. Lateral recumbency is when the animal is held lying on his side.

lateral saphenous The superficial vein that runs along the outside of cats' and dogs' legs.

learned helplessness An emotional state in which the animal has learned through past experience that their behavior does not change the outcome of a circumstance, and therefore they stop trying and shut down.

limbic system This system includes the amygdala, hippocampus, thalamus, hypothalamus, basal ganglia, and cingulate gyrus, which all compose the emotion center of the brain and memory center.

low-restraint animal care The smallest amount of restraint is used to be effective and still not stressful to the patient.

lure-reward training A type of animal training where the animal follows a reinforcer into position and then is given the treat.

M

marker-based training A form of animal training where the correct behavior is marked with a bridging stimulus, such as a clicker or a whistle, and then reinforced.

metacommunication Nonverbal cues, such as body language, that carry meanings that either enhance or dismiss what is being said.

midline A median line or plane that separates the body into two symmetrical parts.

N

need A veterinary procedure that must be performed to save the life of an animal.

negative punishment Subtraction of a pleasurable stimulus to decrease the likelihood an animal will perform a behavior again.

negative reinforcement Subtraction of an aversive stimulus to increase the likelihood an animal will perform a behavior again.

neutral stimulus Anything that has an effect on behavior before conditioning occurs.

no-restraint animal care A progressive form of animal care where no restraint is used by a team member. Instead, team members analyze body language and comfort level, and the animal is free to move away if nervous.

NPO Latin *nil per os*, which means "nothing through the mouth." In medicine, NPO means to withhold food and water.

O

olfaction The process of odorants binding to specific receptors located in the nasal cavity, creating the sense of smell.

operant conditioning (also called *Skinnerian conditioning* or *instrumental conditioning*) A method of learning through trial and error that creates associations between behavior and consequence.

operant counterconditioning (also called *response substitution*) A form of behavior modification performed by changing the animal's behavioral response from an unwanted behavior to a desired behavior in response to the same stimuli.

P

palpation Examination using hands to feel the organs and check for masses.

panniculus response A skin flinch reflex that occurs as a response to evaluation of the spinal column by pressing bilaterally along the spine.

parasympathetic nervous system A portion of the involuntary nervous system responsible for slowing the heart rate and increasing digestion and glandular activity.

patient-centered treatment A method of practicing medicine where the whole patient, mind and body, is treated. This method focuses on reducing stress and fear in the hospital environment as well as home environment.

perception The process of receiving and interpreting information from sensory organs.

pheromones A chemical substance produced by animals and released into the environment to leave "messages" for others of the same species. These messages can have a behavioral impact on the receiver.

piloerection Involuntary bristling of hairs due to cold, shock, or fright due to the stimulation of sympathetic nerves.

pinna The outer flap of the ear.

positive punishment Addition of an aversive stimulus to decrease the likelihood an animal will perform a behavior again.

positive reinforcement Addition of a pleasurable stimulus to increase the likelihood an animal will perform a behavior again.

primary reinforcer Anything that the learner finds inherently reinforcing and that needs no associations with another reinforcer (like a secondary reinforcer).

procedure-centered treatment An approach to practicing medicine where the main focus is completion of procedures and not consideration of the stress or fear level of the patient.

punishment Anything that decreases behavior.

pupillary light response (PLR) A test performed by shining a light into one eye and watching to make sure both pupils constrict.

R

radiographs An image of the inside of an animal created when x-rays pass through the animal to a film cassette or digital sensor.

rate of reinforcement The number of reinforcers an animal receives in one minute's time.

recumbency Lying down.

reflex Involuntary response of an organism.

reinforcement Anything that increases behavior.

response substitution See *Operant counterconditioning.*

restraint Physically holding an animal, usually in certain positions so they cannot flee.

rod A light-sensing cell in the retina of the eye responsible for monochromic vision in poor light.

S

sclera The white outer layer of the eye.

sensation Input from the five senses vision, hearing, smell, touch, and taste.

sensitization After repeated exposure to a stimulus, the animal has a progressively amplified response.

sensory organs The five organs responsible for sensation: eyes, ears, nose, skin, and tongue. The vomeronasal organ is also a sensory organ.

shaping Teaching a new behavior through selectively reinforcing small criteria toward the desired behavior.

shock A life-threatening condition that causes a drop in blood pressure, creating inadequate blood flow to vital organs.

socialization The process of learning to behave in a socially acceptable way. In dog training, it refers to the act of exposing young puppies and kittens to novel people, objects, handling, noises, and other sensations in a positive way.

sternal Pertaining to the sternum, also known as the breastbone. Sternal recumbency is when an animal is held in the "down" position and is resting on the sternum.

stifle Knee joint of the dog or cat.

stimulus control The predictability of a behavior performed in the presence of a stimulus (see "Stimulus Control" in the Appendix for more information).

stress Mental or emotional strain. Stress can be *chronic*, which is over a long period of time, or *acute*, which is a short amount of time like at the veterinary hospital.

subcutaneous Under the skin, such as with subcutaneous injection where the medication or vaccine is injected under the skin layer.

T

tapetum lucidum The reflector portion of the eyes of dogs and cats. This reflector allows the light-sensitive retinal cells to receive more photoreceptor stimulation.

target An object or a piece of the trainer's body that the animal should place a piece of their body to.

thoracic inlet The upper boundary of the thoracic cavity and where the jugular vein is occluded for venipuncture.

three-term contingency Smallest unit of behavioral analysis; this process relies on analyzing behavior through antecedents, behavior, and consequences.

trainer Someone who works to change behavior in animals. Currently, there are no governing bodies over animal trainers.

training plan A written plan of the steps a trainer may need to take to achieve a goal behavior when working with a specific animal. Training plans may also consist of environmental management, reinforcer preference, and shaping plans (see the Appendix for training plans).

trigger stacking Where many stressors that cause an emotional response by the animal accumulate, causing an emotional outburst.

U

unconditioned stimulus Anything that elicits a reaction from an animal without prior conditioning.

V

vasovagal A response to stress (including emotional or physical stress) that involves overactivity of the vagus nerve, sometimes resulting in a drop in blood pressure as well as fainting.

venipuncture The puncturing of a vein; also called a *blood draw* or *intravenous access*.

veterinary behaviorist A veterinarian who has completed a residency in behavior and passed the boarding examination given by the American College of Veterinary Behaviorists.

veterinary technician (RVT, LVT, or CVT) An individual who has met the criteria to work as a veterinary technician in their state.

veterinary technician specialist in behavior (VTS Behavior) A licensed veterinary technician who has met the qualifications and passed the examination given by the Academy of Veterinary Behavior Technicians.

vibrissae Specialized long, stiff whiskers that grow around the face; used as organs of touch.

vomeronasal organ (VNO) Chemoreceptor tubes that are connected to the oral and nasal cavity. The VNO is tied to the limbic system, which is the emotion center of the brain.

W

want A veterinary procedure that a team member or owner would like to perform on an animal.

Index

Cooperative Veterinary Care, First Edition. Alicea Howell and Monique Feyrecilde.
© 2018 John Wiley & Sons, Inc. Published 2018 by John Wiley & Sons, Inc.
Companion website: www.wiley.com/go/howell/cooperative